Where Lt. Colonel Weinstein has been featured:

Fitness Magazine
The History Channel
Fox Sports Net
Fox News Channel - Fox & Friends
The Washington Times
The Las Vegas Tribune
Eurosport TV
Gold Coast Magazine
Tropical Life Magazine Miami
The Sun-sentinel South Florida
The Miami Herald
USA Today
Oxygen Magazine
Univision
Telemundo
RAZOR Magazine
Boca Raton Magazine
Comcast Newsmakers
Army Times
Go Riverwalk Fort Lauderdale
WSFL The Morning Show
NBC Nonstop Miami
NBC6 South Florida Today
New Times Broward-Palm Beach
Navy League News - Fort Lauderdale Council
The Navy Leaguer
SoBeFit Magazine

"Whatever women do they must do twice as well as men to be thought half as good. Luckily, this is not difficult."
— Charlotte Whitton

BOOT CAMP

FOR

WOMEN

Hips, Thighs, Butt, Triceps, Abs and More.
Strong and Confident.

Bob Weinstein
Lt. Colonel, U.S. Army, Retired
Boot Camp Fitness Instructor

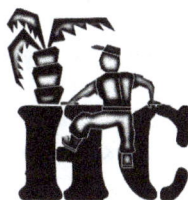

Health Colonel Publishing
www.BeachBootCamp.net

Colonel Bob's Blog:
ColonelBobsBeachBootCamp.blogspot.com/

Boot Camp for Women: Hips, Thighs, Butt, Triceps, Abs and More.
Strong and Confident.
By Bob Weinstein, Lt. Colonel, US Army, Retired.
Note: Bob is the nickname of Lt. Colonel Joseph R. Weinstein, US Army, Ret.
www.BeachBootCamp.net
Categories: physical fitness, boot camp fitness, boot camp workouts

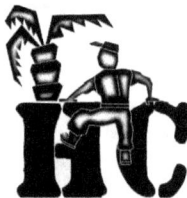

Health Colonel Publishing

ISBN-13: 978-1-935759-20-1
ISBN-10: 1-935759-20-5
Library of Congress Control Number: 2013908149

Before beginning any exercise program, consult your physician. The author and publisher of this book and workout disclaim any liability, personal or professional, resulting from the misapplication of any of the training instructions described in this publication.

Weinstein, Bob.
Boot Camp for Women: Hips, Thighs, Butt, Triceps, Abs and More.
Strong and Confident.
/ by Bob Weinstein, Lt. Colonel, US Army, Ret..– 1st ed.
ISBN-13: 978-1-935759-20-1 (trade pbk. : alk. Paper)
1. Fitness, Exercise –United States. I. Weinstein, Bob. Weinstein, Joseph.
II. Title. III. Boot Camp for Women

Printed in the United States

BOOT CAMP
FOR
WOMEN

Hips, Thighs, Butt, Triceps, Abs and More.
Strong and Confident.

Bob Weinstein
Lt. Colonel, U.S. Army, Retired
Boot Camp Fitness Instructor

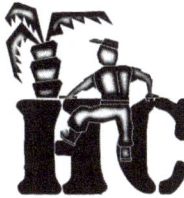

Health Colonel Publishing
www.BeachBootCamp.net

Colonel Bob's Blog:
ColonelBobsBeachBootCamp.blogspot.com/

"The successful person makes a habit of doing what the failing person doesn't like to do."

- Thomas Edison

ACKNOWLEDGEMENTS

Many thanks to all the
beach boot camp recruits on Fort Lauderdale Beach.
You remain a constant source of inspiration.
I thank you for your friendship and camaraderie.
May you prosper and enjoy a healthy and happy life.
I thank the Harbor Beach Marriott Resort & Spa on Fort
Lauderdale Beach in South Florida
for allowing me to use their property.
A special thank you goes to my wife, Grit,
who supports me in all that I do. Thank you to TJ
Gillespie for the great photos. Thank you Darlene
Wooldridge, Katerina Kostioukhina, Merisia Challenger
and Grit Weinstein for your great job posing for the
exercises.

Photography by TJ Gillespie
www.DreamingInPhotography.com

I've got a woman's ability to stick to a job and get on with it when everyone else walks off and leaves it.

— Margaret Thatcher

TABLE OF CONTENTS

TABLE OF CONTENTS

TABLE OF CONTENTS

INTRODUCTION

In the past ten years I have found that women lead the way when it comes to any form of group exercise. That is the reason for the focus on women and boot camp. The mission of this boot camp book for women is health, not combat, not glamour and not appearance although a fit person always looks better and is generally in a better mood and less stressed. This is your opportunity to exercise your complete body without ever stepping into a gym or the need for any expensive gym equipment.

You will find natural body weight, military-style exercises as well as other useful exercises with the dumbbells, the Swiss ball and the resistance band. Your approach to physical fitness should always be a complete body workout to include the cardio. I have included a section on 15 minute workouts designed to work the cardio and complete body strength while maximizing your calorie burn.

Maintain a complete body approach and always be health focused when exercising. And, by the way, keep it fun.

Bob Weinstein
Lt. Colonel, U.S. Army, Retired
www.beachbootcamp.net

HOW TO USE THIS BOOK

Some of the exercises in this book are for all fitness levels, others are more advanced. Some of the more advanced exercises can be safely modified while you develop your muscles to be able to complete the full range of motion. Use the workout plans and seek out a workout buddy to help keep you on track.

You do not need a group environment to perform any of these exercises. All you need is the determination to get started and stay at it. You do not want to belong to that club called "regret" after many years from now because you did not take care of your most important asset, your health. I am certain you will find the time since I know you have 24 hours available per day. Interruptions in your workout routine will happen from time to time. Make sure that any interruption of your workout routine is of a temporary nature. That is a decision that you make and not one that is dictated by the circumstances.

Staying fit and healthy is a long-term goal, not one that comes and goes based on how you feel. A health-focused exercise program is not the same as a more advanced athletic program or one that focuses on appearance. Make sure that you are adjusting your lifestyle to include exercise, healthy eating and healthy thoughts so that you may more fully enjoy life and have more energy to help others and work more productively.

A woman's guess is much more accurate than a man's certainty.
— Rudyard Kipling

PART A

BASIC BOOT CAMP INFO

GROUND RULES TO SUCCEED

1. Know the who, what, why, how, when and where.
Get your plan together and don't worry if it is incomplete. Action is preceded by planning. Some of the details of that goal are gathered while you are on the move to achieve your goals. This serves the purpose of helping you to keep the who, what, why, how, when and where covered as you pursue your journey to better health. A poem by Rudyard Kipling says it best:

> *"I keep six honest serving-men*
> *(They taught me all I knew.)*
> *Their names are What and Why and When*
> *And How and Where and Who."*

2. Never give up if the cause is worthy.
Better health is a worthy cause. Therefore, never ever give up. Sir Winston Churchill said it best:
"Never give in--never, never, never, never, in nothing great or small, large or petty, never give in except to convictions of honour and good sense."
3. Go around, through, over or under all obstacles.
There will be obstacles along the way. Deal with them and overcome them. There will be interruptions, set-backs, and thoughts of "I don't feel like it." that will invade the mind.
4. Inject Vitamin "D" for Discipline into your plan.
Include a good dose of D for discipline to keep you on track when you don't feel like it.
5. Take personal responsibility for your situation.
Never blame external circumstances or other people. That will keep you empowered to improve.

GOALS - THREE-STEP ACTION PLAN

1. Acknowledge and RECOGNIZE that there is a problem.

Have your "deviant" eating habits and lack of exercise become a lifestyle? Acknowledging and recognizing the problem appears to be easy to accomplish. It is easy because there is no action required other than acknowledgement and recognition. As Albert Einstein once said, *"Insanity is doing the same thing over and over again and expecting a different result."* If we are acknowledging and recognizing the problem with the forethought that no action is required, it is bogus and does not count. It is not genuine. Motives do matter and the motive with forethought that no action is required will not bring about the positive change you are looking for.

2. DECIDE when and how you are going to take action.

Decide when you will start and how you will take action.

3. Take ACTION.

Get up and start working on your goals now. Get up in the morning and start writing down all that you eat and drink. Write down your exercising routines. Move and allow momentum to overcome inertia.

WORLD RECORD WOMEN

There are many categories of women's world record athletic events.

50 Meters in 5.93+ seconds: Marion Jones from the United States in 1999.

100 Meters in 10.49 seconds. Florence Joyner from the United States made this world record in 1988.

200 Meters in 21.34 seconds: Florence Joyner, 1988.

400 Meters in 47.60 seconds: Marita Koch from former East Germany in 1985.

Mile Run in 4:12.56: Svetlana Masterkova from Russia achieved this record time for a one mile run in 1996.

Half Marathon in 1:05:50: Mary Keitany from Kenya in 2011.

Marathon in 2:15:25: Paula Radcliffe from Great Britain in 2003.

MYTHS ABOUT EXERCISE

There are many myths about women and exercises. Here are just a few of them:

Myth #1: Isolate the muscle for best results.

Muscles are best worked in orchestration. That means pick multi joint exercises such as push-ups, squats or lunges.

Myth #2: Working the abs will reduce belly fat.

No. Working the abs will not reduce belly fat. You cannot spot reduce any body part.

Myth #3: Muscle can turn to fat if you stop working out.

Muscle cannot turn to fat and fat cannot turn to muscle. You will add fat because your body has excess calories it did not burn or you may be stressed and your body stores extra fat as an emergency measure.

Myth #4: Never eat before a workout.

Always eat something before a workout, preferably carbs. That will increase your energy and enhance your performance which will improve your fitness gain.

Myth #5: A good sweat will increase weight loss.

A good sweat is a good sweat and will not result in weight loss. If the real source of your sweat is because you are working out, you are probably burning more calories. If your sweat is a result of the sauna you just lost lots of water and some electrolytes.

US ARMY FITNESS TEST

How do you measure up according to military standards as a woman? The fitness test chart below will let you know how you stand. The US Army requires that soldiers achieve a minimum score of at least 60% after basic training. Some elite units have higher standards. To test yourself correctly, you have two minutes for each event, push-ups and sit-ups to complete as many as you can. The 2-mile run is to be completed as fast as you can. The age groups 27 - 31 and 32 - 36 are depicted with passing scores.

Age	Gender	Push-ups	Sit-ups	2-mile Run
27 - 31	Male	39	45	17:00
27 - 31	Female	17	45	20:30
32 - 36	Male	36	42	17:42
32 - 36	Female	15	42	21:42

WOMEN IN COMBAT

In February 2013 the decision has been made to allow women in combat. Are you combat material? You may not have to ask yourself this question if you are not interested in a combat position. However, if you are a woman presently serving on active duty in a non-combat role, there may be battlefield circumstances where you will find yourself ordered into a combat role although this was never your intent as a woman in the military.

According to the Pentagon, as of January 2013 there are 1.4 million men and women serving on active duty in the military. Of those, 237,000 are in combat positions.

The standards for a combat position in the military will purportedly be gender neutral. For non-combat positions there are two standards for the physical fitness tests, one for women and one for men. For our elite forces, such as Navy SEALS, Army Rangers and other special forces, there will probably be exemptions which means that women may not be allowed. By the way, very few men make it successfully through the rigorous training.

MUSCLE CHART

MAJOR MUSCLE GROUPS

The Major Skeletal Muscles of the Human Body

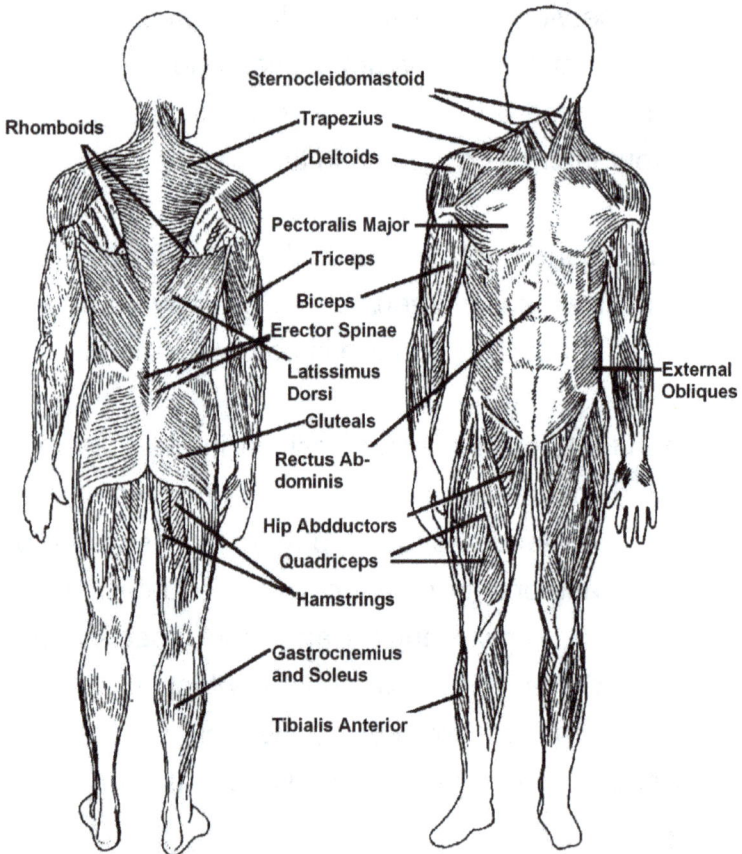

Rhomboids

Sternocleidomastoid

Trapezius

Deltoids

Pectoralis Major

Triceps

Biceps

Erector Spinae

Latissimus Dorsi

Gluteals

Rectus Ab-dominis

Hip Abdductors

Quadriceps

Hamstrings

Gastrocnemius and Soleus

Tibialis Anterior

External Obliques

The iliopsoas muscle (a hip flexor) cannot be seen as it lies beneath other muscles. It attaches to the lumbar, the pelvis, the vertebrae and the femur.

EXERCISE AS PHYSICAL THERAPY

Consider physical exercise as a form of physical therapy. Exercise is considered the best way to treat back problems and disk injury according to Consumer Medical Reports. Although I have lower back and shoulder injuries from the past, as long as I am exercising, I have no pain and no issues. My personal exercise consists mostly of running and natural body weight exercises and in many cases I combine the run with intermittent body weight exercises. Stay in touch with your body to make sure you are not injuring yourself by exercising and consult with your doctor before you start your exercise program, especially if you have prior injuries.

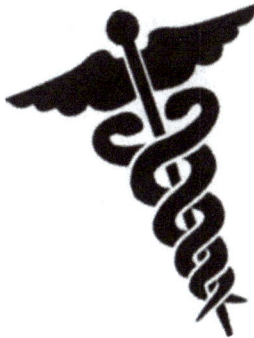

PAIN

Maintaining a balance of complete body exercises combined with cardio is a great way to reduce the chance of injury or pain. Muscle soreness due to a workout is not pain and it is best to continue your workout routine and simply go easier on the exercises instead of taking rest days. This approach is called active recovery. That will promote a quicker and healthier recovery. The most important rule here is to listen to your body. If you find that you genuinely feel pain and it does not go away after a few days, you should see your doctor and follow his or her advice.

You may have certain injuries from the past that require you to modify certain exercises. Work around your old injuries and you will still be able to take care of your health with a workout program. Seek the advice of your doctor for appropriate exercises and appropriate modification of exercises.

DOES FORM MATTER?

As a general rule, exercise form does matter. Focus on proper form is designed to maximize the use of those muscles which are to be worked for a particular exercise and to maintain good body mechanics. Sometimes, maintaining proper form has the further purpose of preventing injury.

There is, however, a greater principle than form that needs to be applied. That principle is movement. Movement is more important than form as long as you are not injuring yourself. Most body weight exercises can be safely modified. In some cases, modifying an exercise is done to prevent injury. For example, if someone has problems with their knees, it may be advisable to modify the squat so that injury does not occur. Modifying the squat by only performing a partial motion would then allow for continuous work of the muscles without injury.

Many who attend my beach boot camp classes cannot perform regular push-ups. I recommend partial push-ups which means starting in the up position but lowering your body partially instead of going all the way down or simply struggle through during each repetition. This allows you to continue strengthening the muscles needed to perform a full range of motion..

CORE STRENGTH IS KEY

A mindset needs to change when it comes to working the core and, in particular, the abdominals. The predominant, false mindset is to think specifically about performing exercises that focus on the abdominal muscles. This mindset is false because all the muscles of the human body move in orchestration. Therefore, any exercise or drill that takes advantage of the complete or predominant orchestration of the muscles, promotes muscle balance and good body mechanics which will help prevent injury when moving the body in activities of daily life, sports and physical activity at work.

Some examples of activities and exercises that work the core::

Running and sprinting
Interval training
Agility training
Squats
Push-ups
Pull-ups
Swimming
Volleyball
Football
Tennis

THE ULTIMATE BOOT CAMP WOMAN

The ultimate boot camp woman is about much more than exercise, fitness, eating right and appearance. She has her life priorities in order of importance. Her daily and long-term decision making is dictated by her priorities, her values. She also allows for mistakes along the way and is willing to learn from them. She understands that time can only be spent and never saved. Therefore, she uses her time wisely. She knows she is on this earth just a short time and keeps things in perspective when stuff happens. To be fair, these values apply to men as well. Here are her values while keeping in mind there are more:

Faith
Golden Rule
Honesty
Dependability
Kindness
Self-less Service
Loyalty
Duty
Honor
Personal Courage
Patience
Controls the Tongue
Does not Gossip

If you want something said, ask a man; if you want something done, ask a woman.
— Margaret Thatcher

EXERCISES FOR WOMEN

Some of the best exercises for women focus on the hips, thighs, triceps, abs and butt. There are several great abdominal and core exercises for women.

Hips.

Lunges and squats work the hips and butt and many more lower body muscles.

Triceps.

The dip exercise is an excellent way to focus on working the triceps.

Thighs.

Lunges and squats will take care of those thighs.

Butt

Lunges and squats will work if you do enough of them. Interval training with short distance running drills will do wonders for the butt because those muscles must work hard when you run.

"Never try to impress a woman, because if you do she'll expect you to keep up the standard for the rest of your life."

                                        —W. C. Fields

PART B

BODY WEIGHT EXERCISES

BURPEES

Works your **complete body**.

Position yourself in the standing position with feet shoulder width apart and arms to your sides. Squat down and with your hands on the floor. Thrust your legs back so that you are now in the push-up position and then thrust them so that you are back in the squat position with hands on the floor. Now jump up as high as you can. That is one rep. I recommend giving the squat thrust a four count for each rep. That will allow you to count each movement.

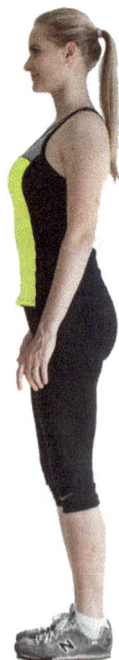

BURPEES

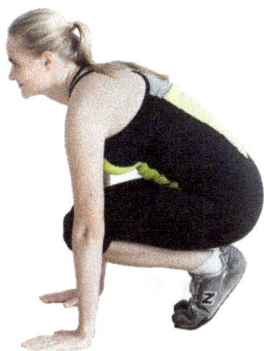

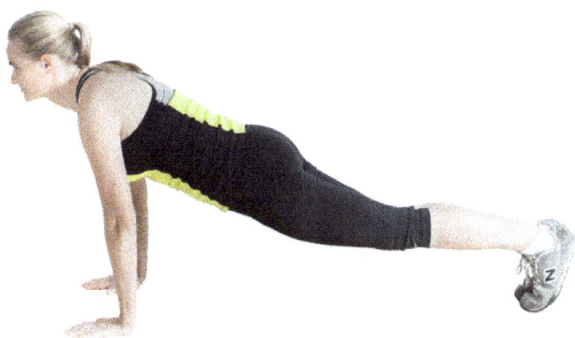

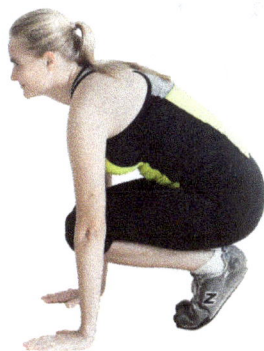

CRUNCHES

Works your **abs and lower back**.

Lie down on your back and bend both knees with your feet on the ground. Clasp your hands behind your head or place them in a crossed position on your chest. Raise your shoulders slightly from the ground and lower them back down. That is one repetition. Perform 1 - 5 sets of 30 to 50 repetitions each.

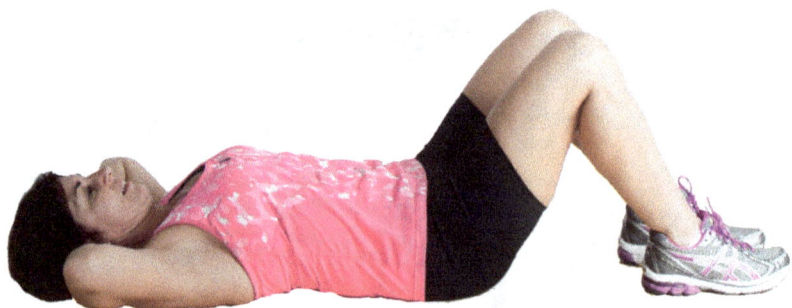

CRUNCHES

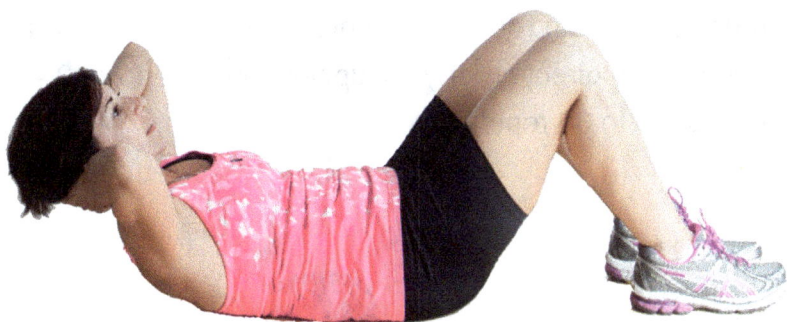

REVERSE CRUNCH

Works your **abs**.

Lie on your back with your knees bent and hands to your sides on the floor or clasped behind your head. While maintaining your knees bent in the 90 degree angle, lift your legs to where your lower legs (from knees to feet) are parallel to the ground. You may increase the reverse crunch by raising your butt while crunching your lower body in the direction of your upper body. Perform 2 - 5 sets of 10 to 30 repetitions.

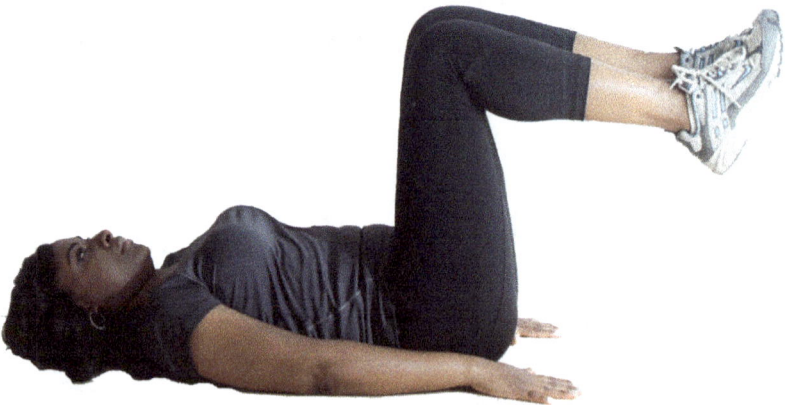

REVERSE CRUNCH

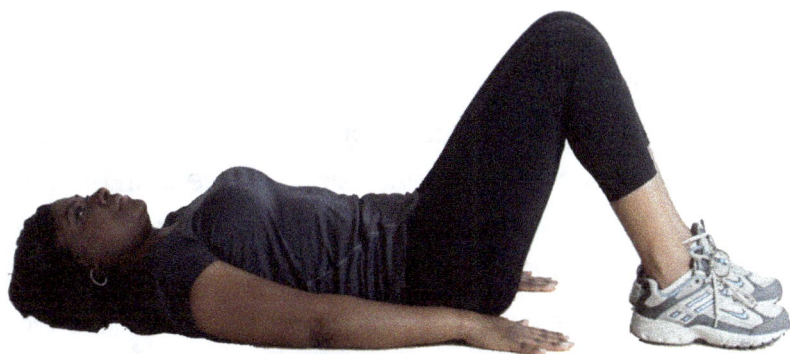

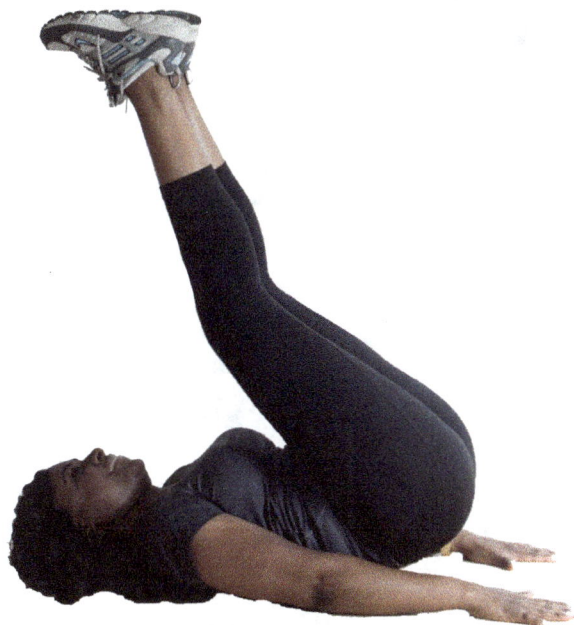

FLUTTER KICKS

Works your **hip flexors, abs and legs**.

Lie on your back with arms extended on the sides of your body and palms facing down on the ground to stabilize the lower back with your head raised. Raise both of your legs in a staggered position (one leg is higher than the other) with a slight bend in the knees. This is a four count exercise. With each count you will simply switch the leg positions which makes it look like a scissor move, not bicycle pedaling. Do five to ten reps per set with multiple sets and very brief rests between sets.

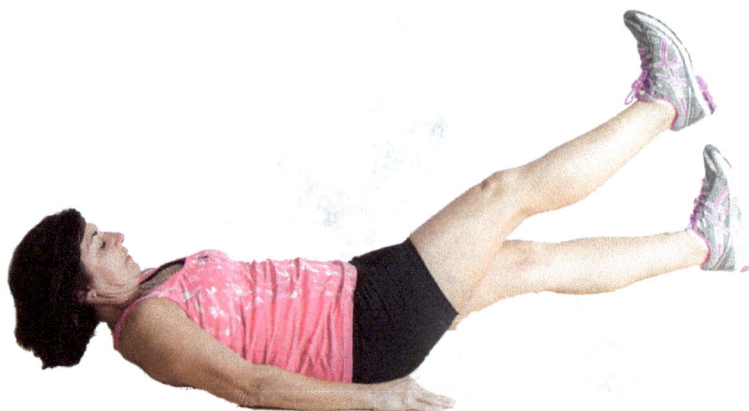

FLUTTER KICKS

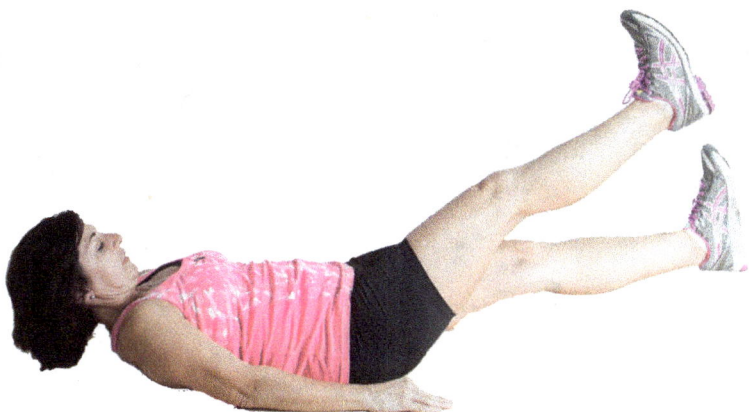

HIGH KICK

Works your **cardio and legs.**

Your right leg is back. Your left leg is forward. Perform a high kick with the right leg by thrusting it out and kicking forward as high as you can and then back to the starting position. That is one repetition. Switch legs to work the other side. For example, if you are performing thirty reps, work first one leg with all thirty and then the other. Count the reps with the leg in the extended (kick) position. Perform 30 to 60 reps with each leg.

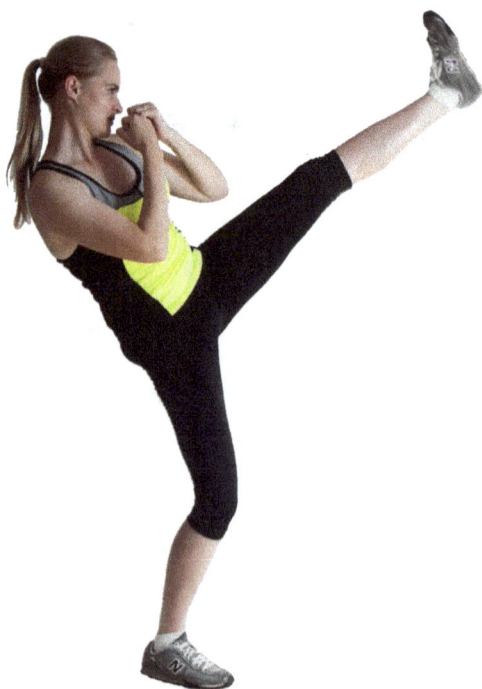

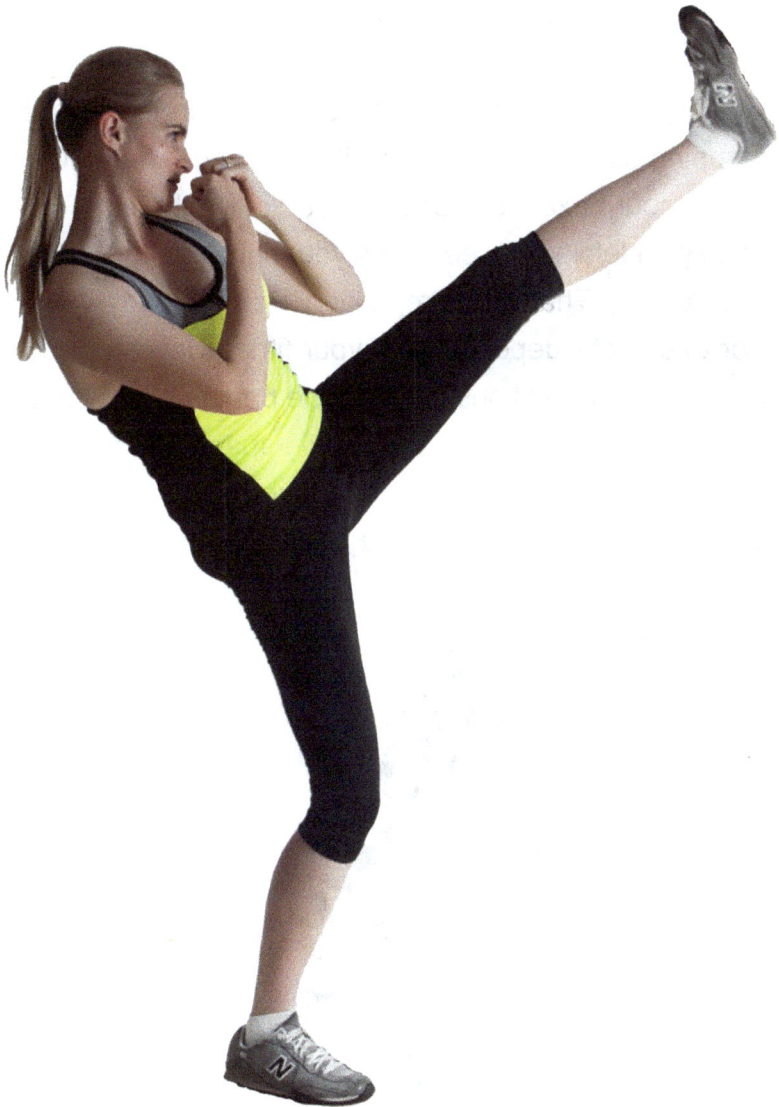

HIGH KICK

HIGH STEP

Works your **cardio and legs and butt.**

Raise your arms up high and begin to run in place by stepping as high as you can with each leg. Treat this as a four-count exercise. One - raise your right leg. Two - raise your left leg. Three - raise your right leg. Four - raise your left leg. That is one repetition. Perform 5 to 10 sets. For each set - depending on your fitness level, perform 20, 30 or 40 repetitions per set. The benefit of this cardio exercise is that it requires very little space and could be performed in a cubicle at work. Maybe you can get your colleagues to join you, cubicle or office room.

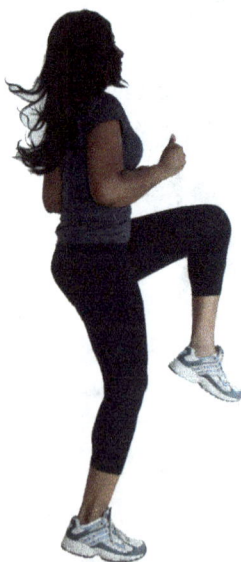

HIGH STEP

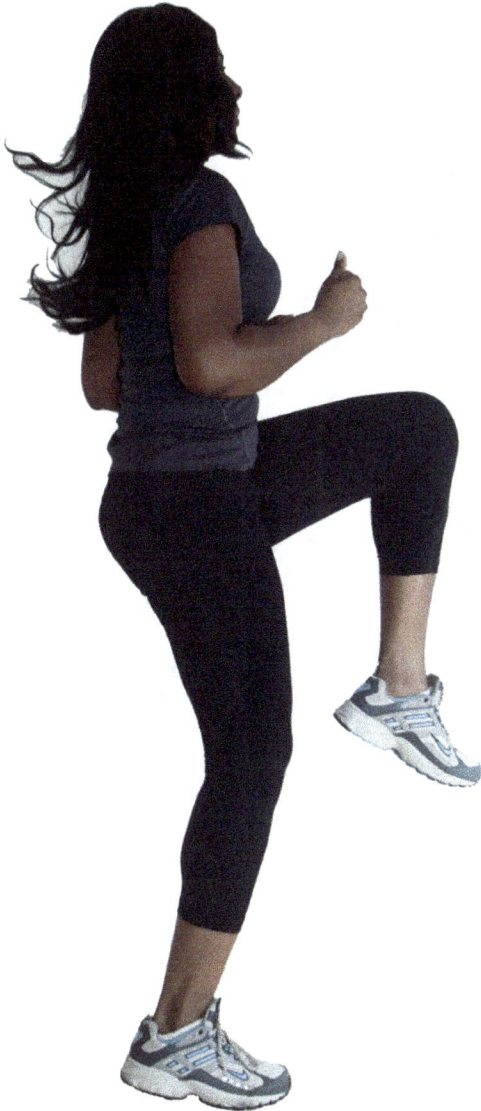

HIP RAISE

Works the **buttocks and core**.

Get down on your back with both knees bent and feet on the floor. Contract your core area; squeeze your buttocks while raising your hips until your body is straight from your knees to your shoulders. Pause for 5 seconds in this position and then lower your body back to the starting position.

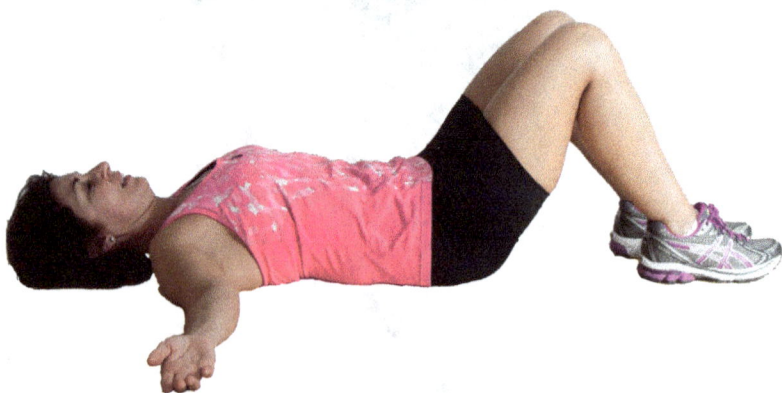

HIP RAISE

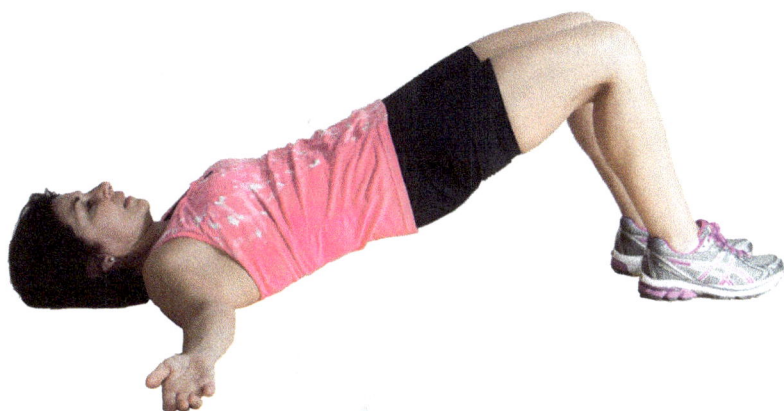

I RAISE

Develops **shoulder strength and stability.**

.

Place your extended arms over your head and parallel to the floor with palms facing each other and thumbs pointing up. Your body is now forming the "I." Raise your arms as high as you can and lower them back down. That is one repetition.

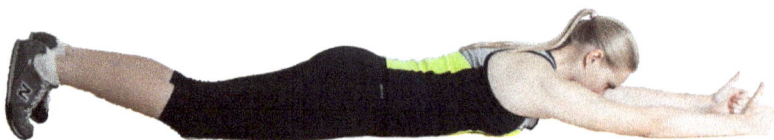

I RAISE

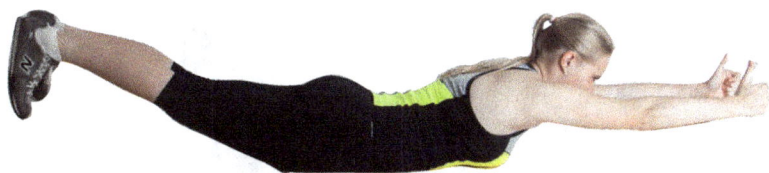

INCLINE PUSHUP

Works the **upper body**.

Get in the push-up position by placing your hands onto an elevated wall or some other very stable object that will support the exercise. You're in the same position as you would be for the standard push-up and you perform them the same way. These are great push-ups for beginners and anyone who may have lower back issues as opposed to performing the standard push-up. Perform 15 to 20 reps per set.

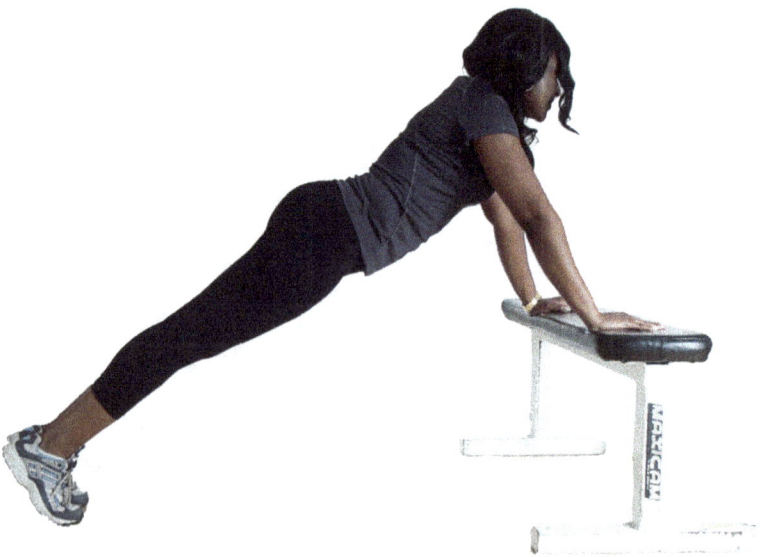

INCLINE PUSHUP

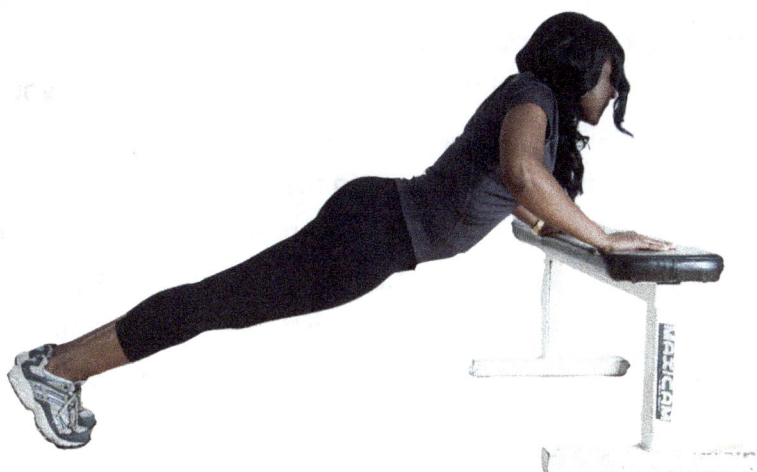

JUMPING JACKS

Works your **cardio and is a warm up exercise.**

A callisthenic workout is never complete without jumping jacks. Stand with feet together and arms at your sides. You're going to need a little bounce for this one. Jump to the spread leg position and land your feet back on the ground while you bring your arms together over your head (arms are raised and extended over your head). Then immediately jump back to the starting position with feet together while bringing your arms back down to your sides. This is a smooth motion. Jump out. Then jump back to the starting position. That is one repetition. Perform 50 to 100 reps. Of course you can start out with less, if you feel the need. This is a high impact exercise. If you have any medical issues with your knees or ankles, please consult your physician. Try modifying the exercise by spreading your legs partially and not jumping as high if you have a medical issue that allows you to modify the exercise.

JUMPING JACKS

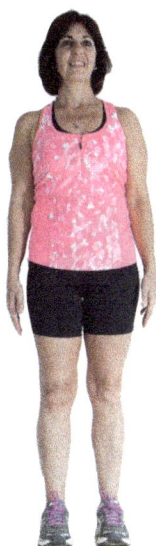

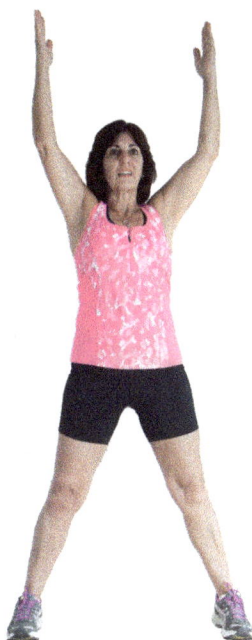

KNEE THRUST

Works the **abs**.

Stand with your right leg forward and a little less than shoulder width apart. Thrust your left knee as close to your chest as possible and back to the starting position with left leg back. That is one rep. You may perform 20 to 40 reps with the same leg and then switch or you can alternate between legs.

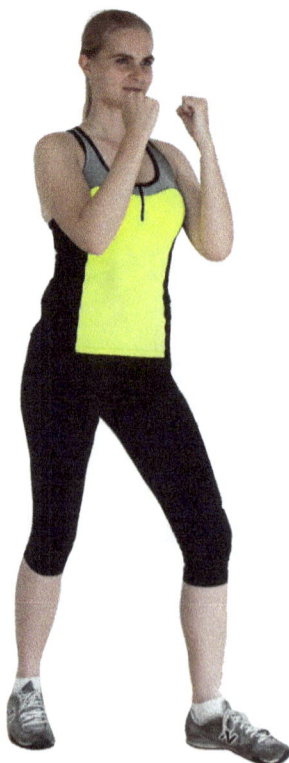

KNEE THRUST

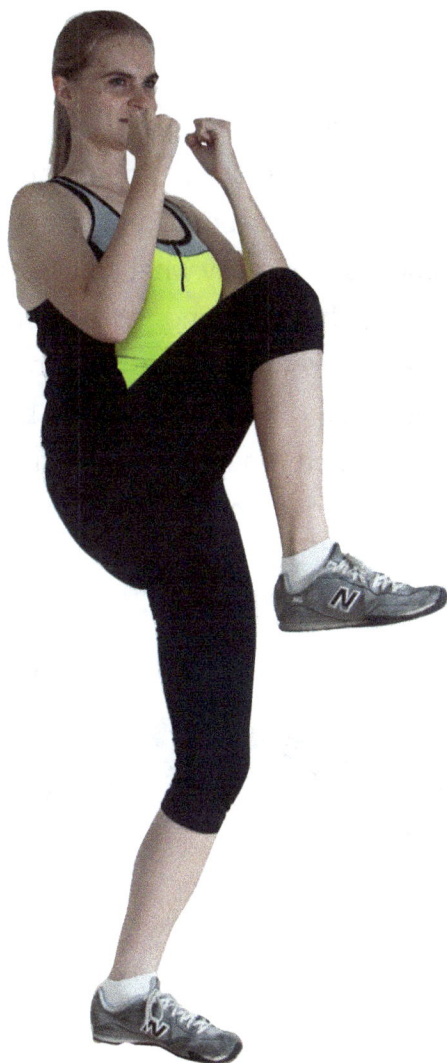

MOUNTAIN CLIMBER.

Works the **butt, hips, legs and thighs.**

Get down in the regular push-up position with arms a little more than shoulder width apart and your body straight. Imagine you are about to go for a run in this position because that is exactly what you are going to do. You will do this by thrusting one leg forward with your knee reaching as close to your chest as possible. Alternate by going for that "run" in the push-up position. Use a count of four for each repetition. Perform 5 to 10 reps per set and more as your fitness progresses.

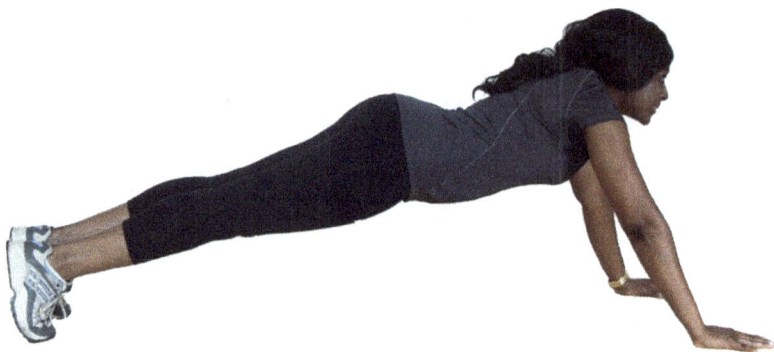

MOUNTAIN CLIMBER.

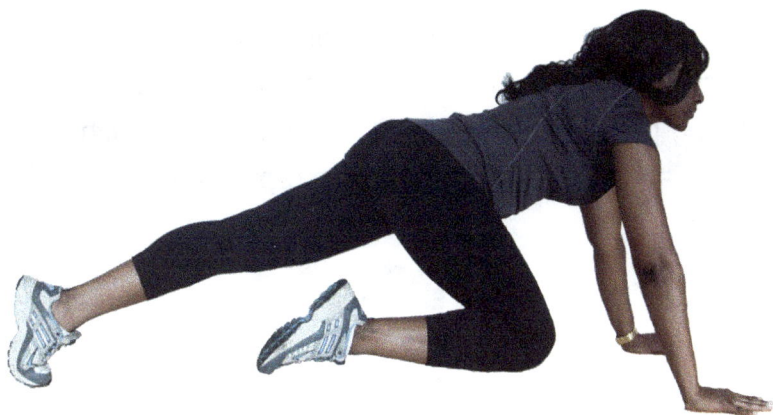

SIDE KICK AND PUNCH

Works **lower body large muscles groups.**

Stand with your feet shoulder width apart and both arms in the guarded position with fists up protecting your face. Bring your right leg up by bending the knee and then thrust the kick out to the right side and then back to the starting position. Then punch straight forward with your left fist and then back. That is one rep.

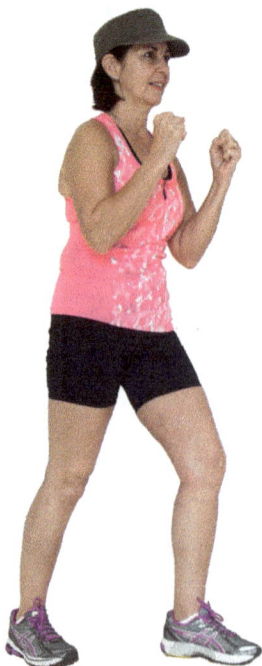

SIDE KICK AND PUNCH

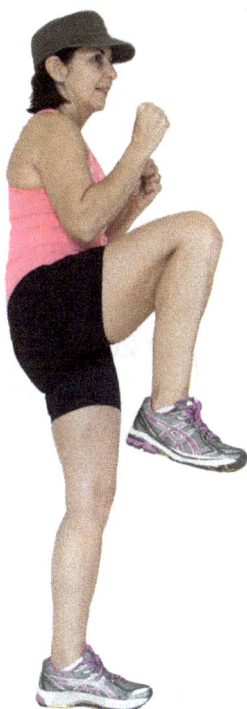

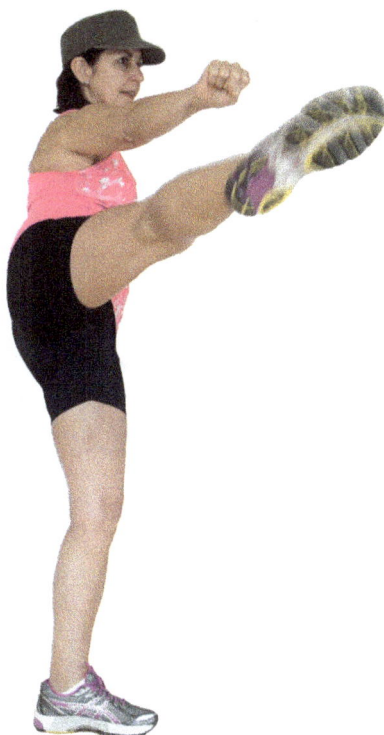

SIDE PLANK

Works the **core muscles.**

Lie on your side on the floor. Place your forearm on the floor under your shoulder and perpendicular to your body. Your legs are extended with your upper leg on top of your lower leg. Raise your body so that it is completely straight and rigid. Hold that position for 20 to 30 seconds or raise and lower your body to perform repetitions. Switch sides and repeat. Perform 10 - 20 repetitions of 3 to 5 sets.

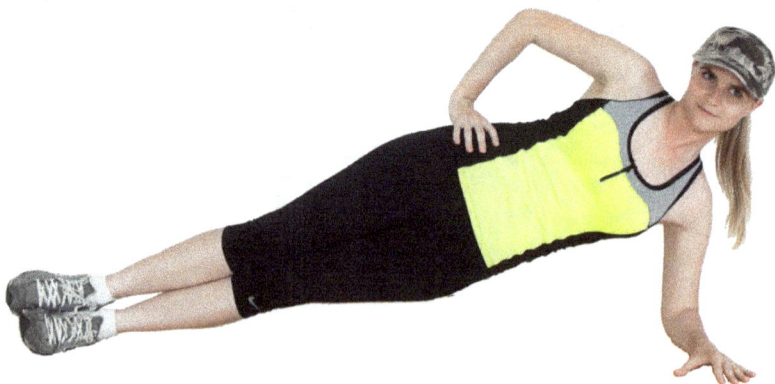

SIDE PLANK

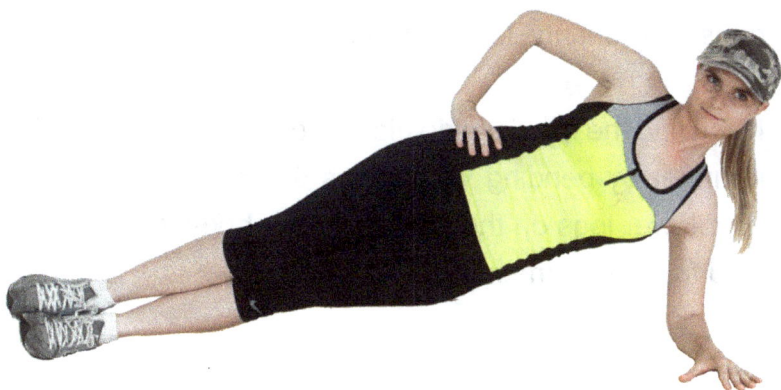

SIDE PLANK MODIFIED

Works the **core muscles.**

If the side plank is too difficult for you, try holding it for just a couple of seconds and then rest for a couple of seconds and continue this until you attain 30 seconds all total.

If you find the regular side plank too difficult, try modifying it further by bending your knees 90 degrees by placing your lower legs on the floor and your body is raised and rigid from your knees up.

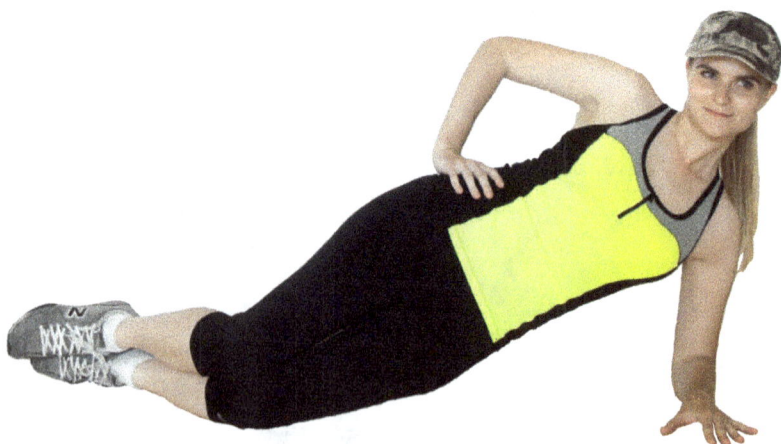

SIDE PLANK MODIFIED

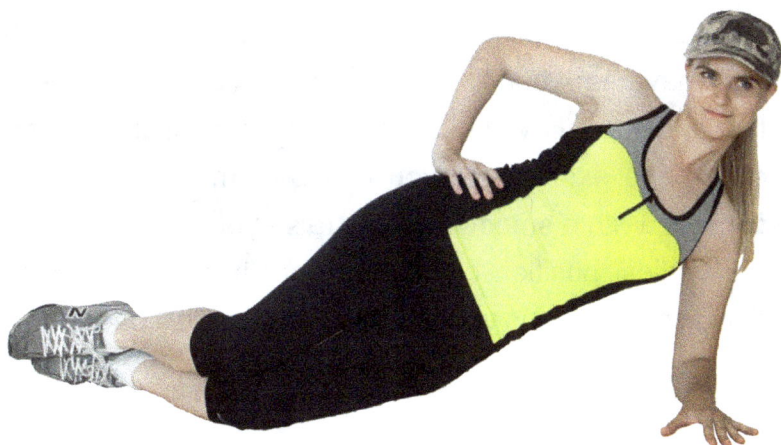

SIT-UPS

Works your **hip flexors and abdominal muscles.**

The sit-up is great for strengthening the abs and hip-flexors. Lie down on your back with your arms across your chest or hands clasped behind your head and knees bent. You may use a buddy to hold your ankles or place your feet under a sturdy object to keep your feet on the ground during the exercise or you can perform it without leg support. With a smooth motion, raise your upper body to the vertical position or beyond and then lower it back down while allowing your spine to roll smoothly back down to the starting position. Perform 3 - 5 sets of 40 to 100 repetitions each.

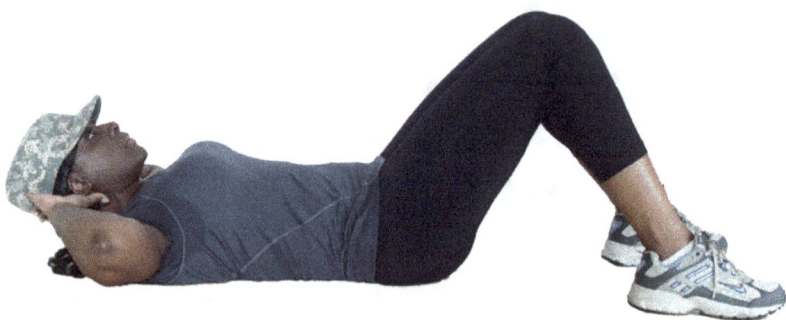

SIT-UPS

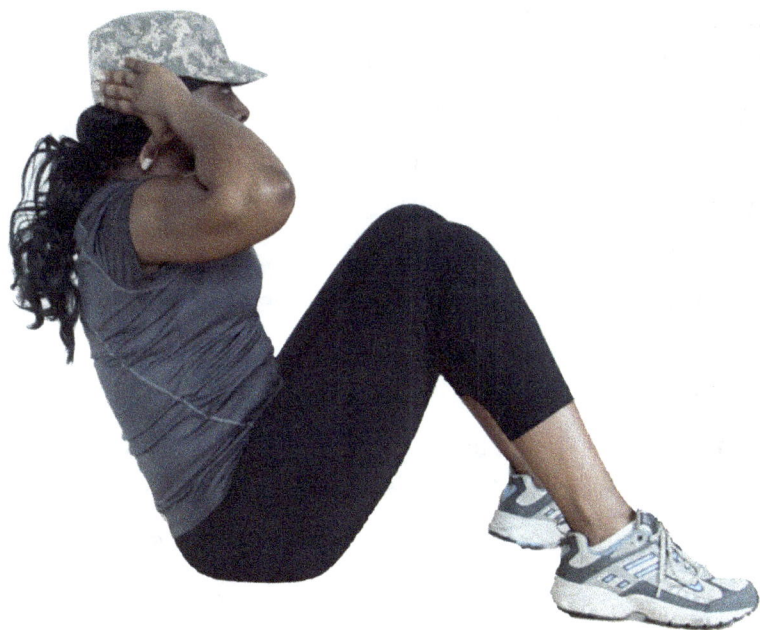

SPIDERMAN PUSHUP

Works the **chest, shoulders, arms and abs.**

Start in the standard push-up position. Use a three count to get all the movements.

Count 1: Bring your body to the down position.

Count 2: Bend your right leg to the side of your body until your knee reaches your right elbow. The right leg remains elevated for this move until it's back to the starting position with foot on the ground.

Count 3: Bring your body back to the standard push-up position.

With the next alternating rep you will use your left leg. Continue your repetitions by alternating between using your right and your left leg for count two. Use the three count to help you stay with the rhythm of the exercise.

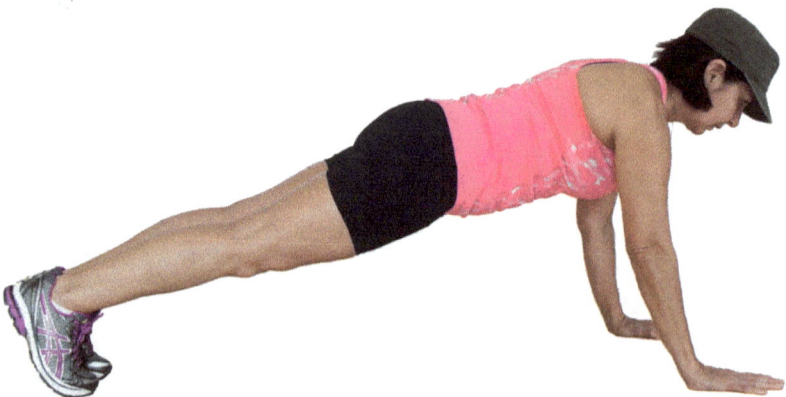

SPIDERMAN PUSHUP

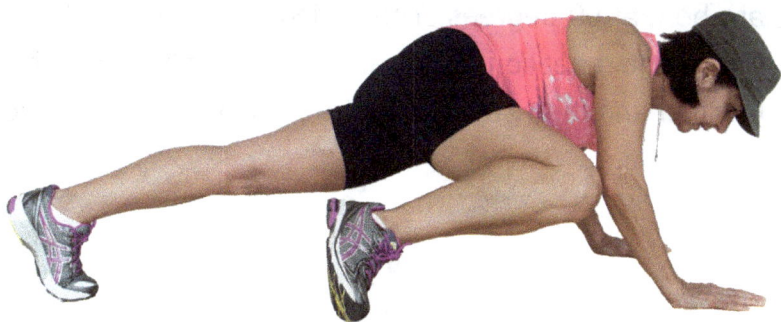

STATIONARY LUNGES

Works the **glutes, butt, hamstrings and quads.**

As with the walking lunge, pretend you are carrying two full buckets of water. Step forward with your right foot to the point where your knees are bent at 90 degrees. Your knee of the forward leg should not go past your big toe. Now simply lower your body to the point where your knees are bent at 90 degrees. Then bring your body back up. That's one repetition. For example, do twenty reps in this position and then switch with the left leg forward and do twenty more.

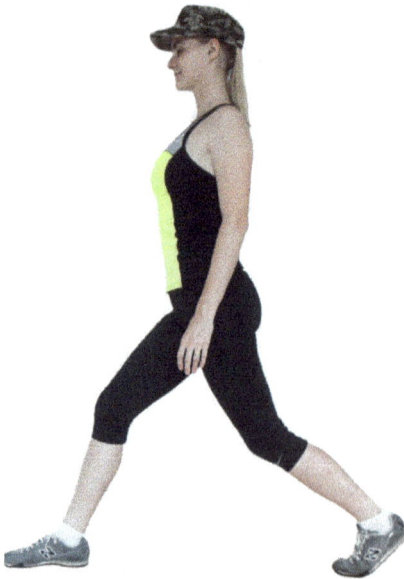

STATIONARY LUNGES

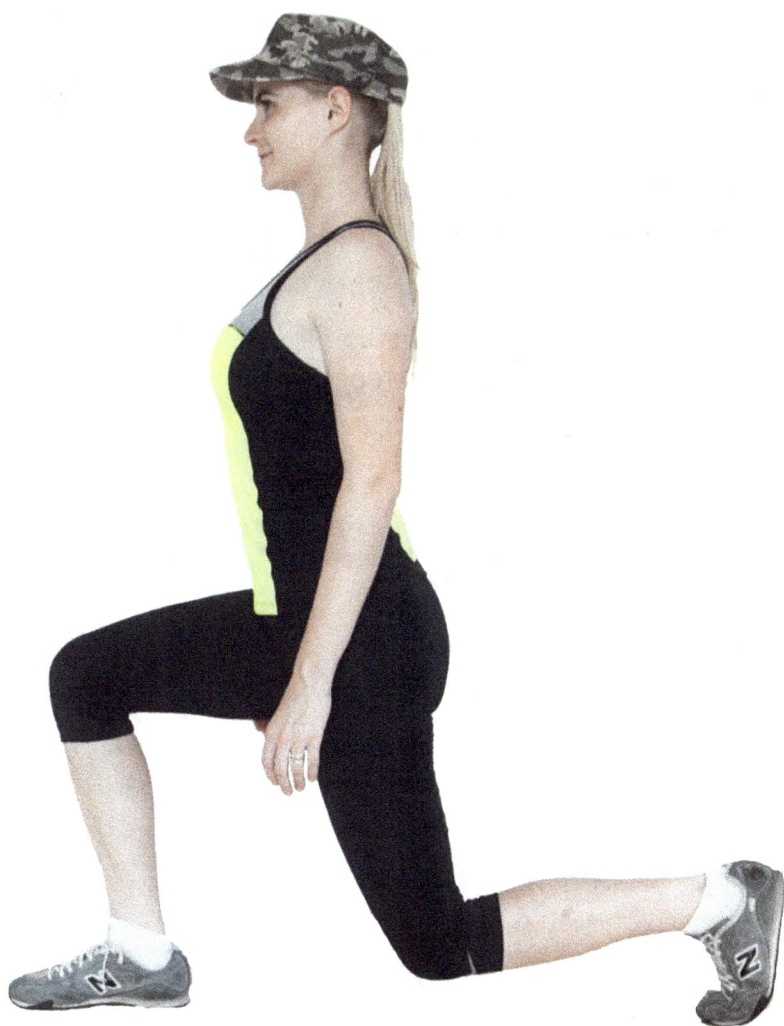

SQUAT

Works the **thighs, hips, butt, quads and hamstrings.**

Your feet are shoulder width apart with your arms on your hips or hands together with elbows bent (or arms extended straight and parallel to the floor) and your head up and upper body in a natural upright position – not the bending over forward ski position. Bend your knees to a 90 degree break making sure that your knee does not go past your big toe. Then bring your body back up to the upright position. That's one repetition.

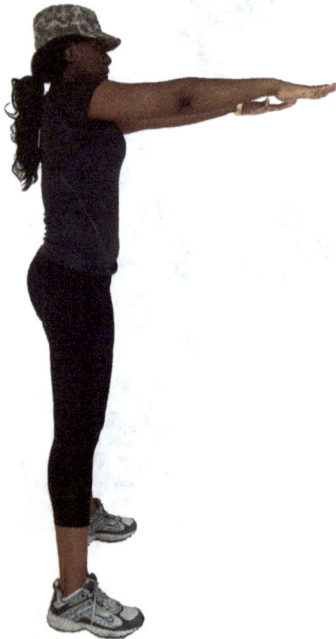

SQUAT

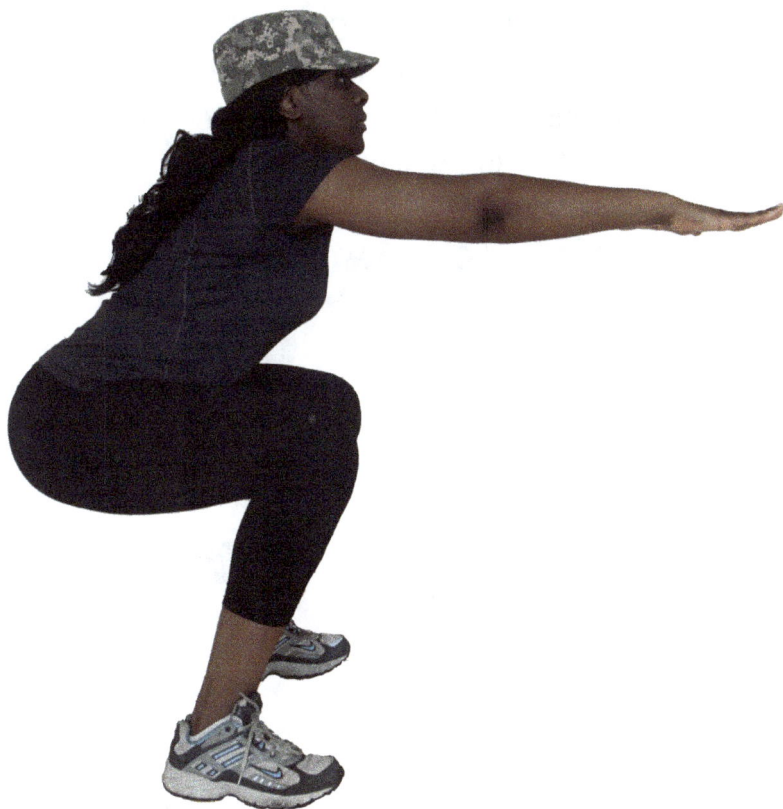

SUPERMAN EXTENSION

Works your **back muscles, lats, traps and glutes.**

Lie down on your stomach and get in the superman flying position with arms and legs extended. Perform one repetition by raising your legs and arms and holding this position for a slow 30 count and then back to the starting position. Perform 3 to 5 sets.

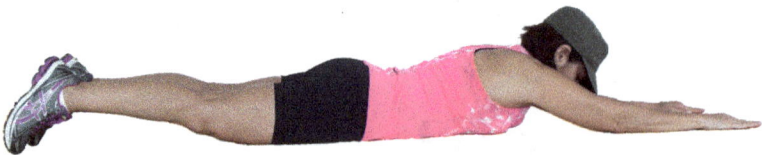

SUPERMAN EXTENSION

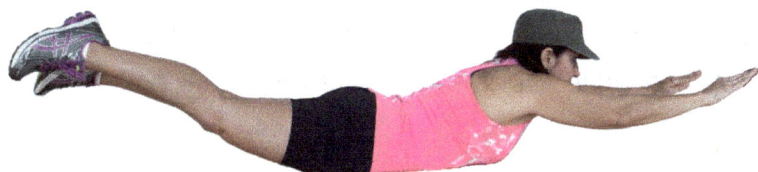

SWIMMER

Works the **shoulders, upper-back, abdominal and hip regions.**

Lie on your stomach with feet and arms together and extended in what looks like a swimming position. Keep your arms and legs straight at all times during the exercise. Move your right arm and left leg up and return to the start position. Then move your left arm and right leg up and return to the start position. Continue the exercise while alternating. Use a moderate rythm.

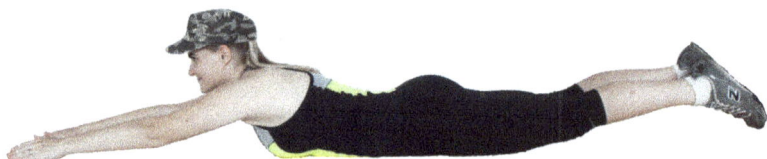

SWIMMER

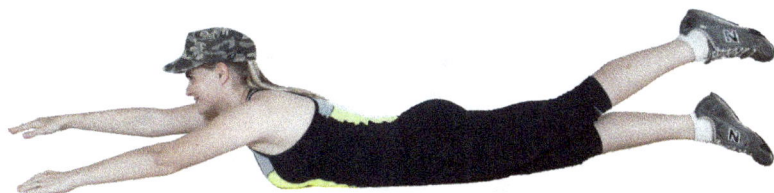

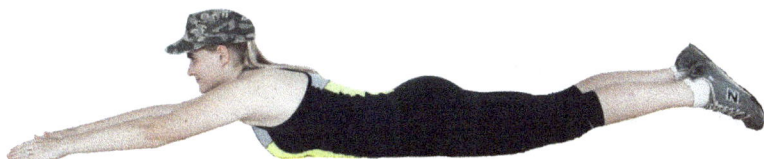

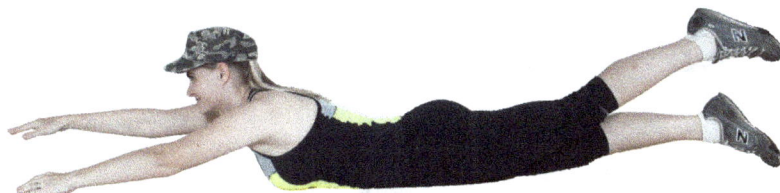

T-PUSHUP

Works **hips, lower back and abs, among other upper body muscles**.

Start in the standard push-up position. Use a three count to get all the movements.
Count 1: Bring your body to the down position.
Count 2: Raise your right arm while turning your body to the side. You left arm is supporting you and is extended. It looks like a T on its side, hence T-Push-up.
Count 3: Bring your body back to the standard push-up position.
With the next alternating rep you will raise your left arm. Continue your repetitions by alternating between using your right and your left arm for count two. Use the three count to help you stay with the rhythm of the exercise.

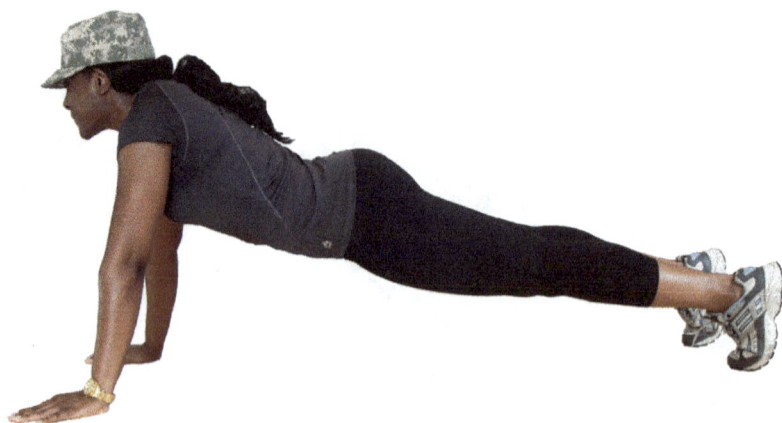

T-PUSHUP

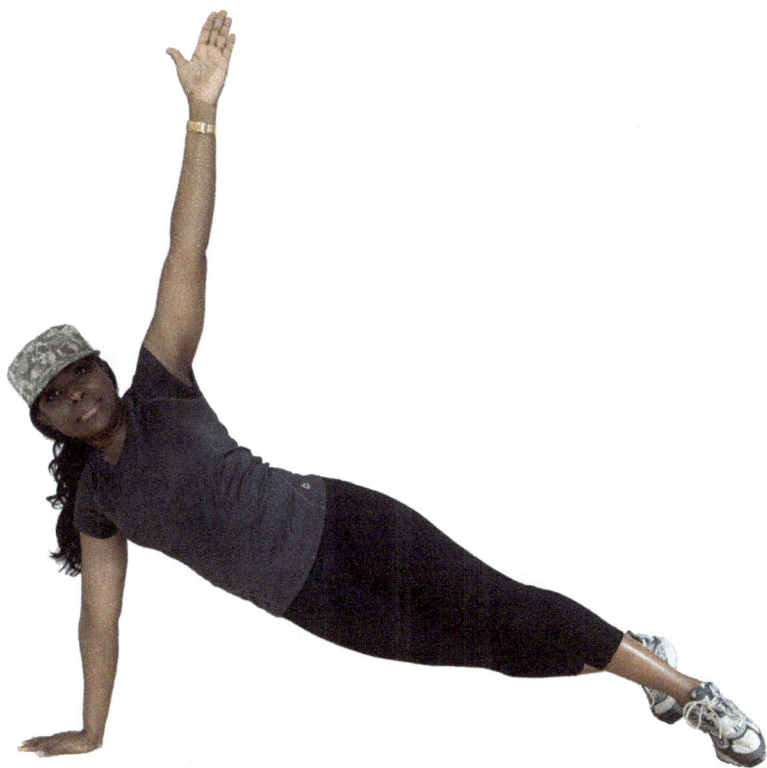

T RAISE

Works the **upper back, rotator cuff, and deltoids.**

The T RAISE is performed just like the Y RAISE except that the arms are extended out to your sides forming a "T." Raise your arms as high as you can and lower them back down. That is one repetition.

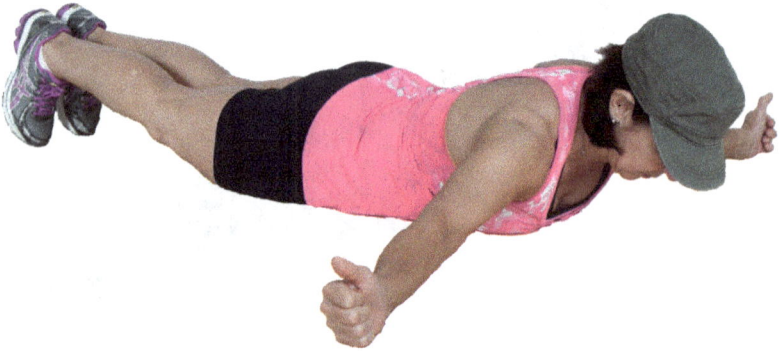

T RAISE

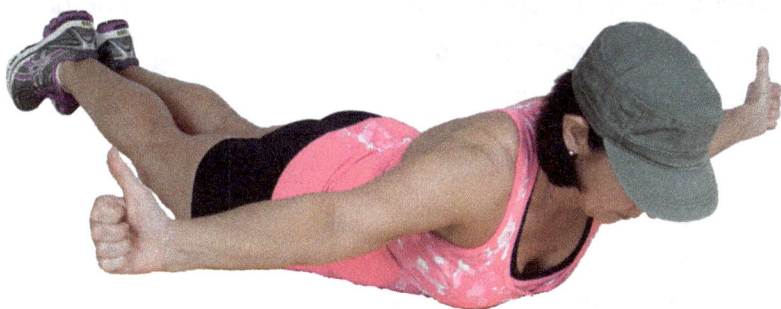

TRICEPS PUSHUPS

Works the **triceps, hips, lower back and abs, among other upper body muscles**.

This time your hands are close together and your feet are spread about shoulder width for stability or your feet may be together if you prefer. Go down to the point where your chest is almost touching the ground and come back up. You'll notice that this one feels more strenuous than the regular push-up.

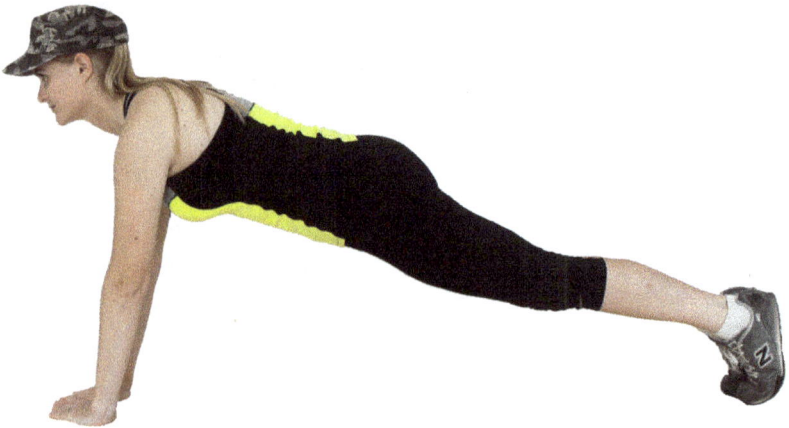

TRICEPS PUSHUPS

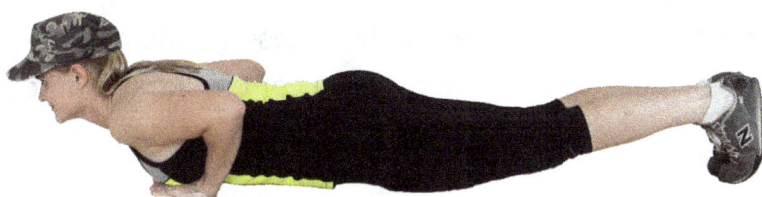

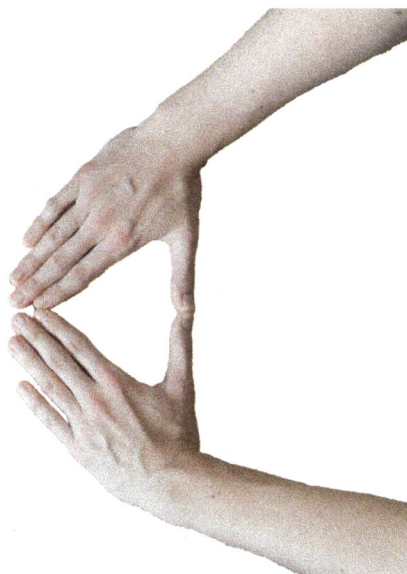

WIDE PUSHUPS

Works the **chest, arms, shoulders and back.**

The wide (extra wide) push-up is performed the same way as the regular push-up with one exception. This time your hands are spread as wide as you can get them without collapsing. Your body is closer to the ground in the starting position. You will notice how the chest now enjoys a very beneficial workout along with your arms.

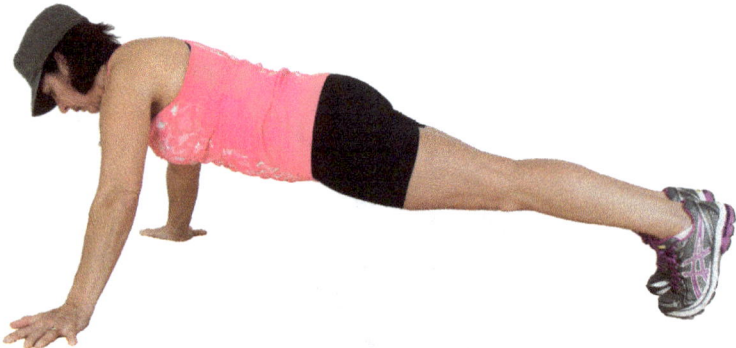

WIDE PUSHUPS

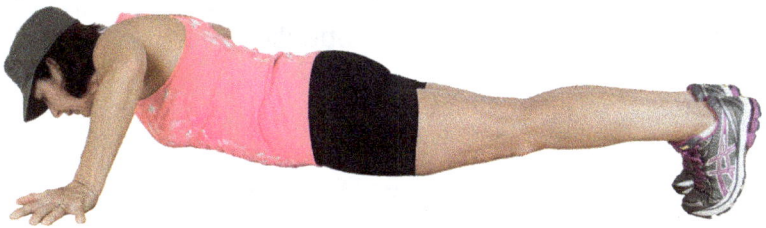

WIND MILLS

Warm-up and flexibility exercise.

Stand with your feet wider than shoulder width apart and arms extended parallel to the ground out to your sides and palms facing down with elbows locked. Bend over and take your right hand diagonally across your body and reach for your left foot while extending your left arm pointing towards the sky and then back to the starting position. In the starting position you are not bent over but standing erect between each repetition. Perform 10 to 20 reps.

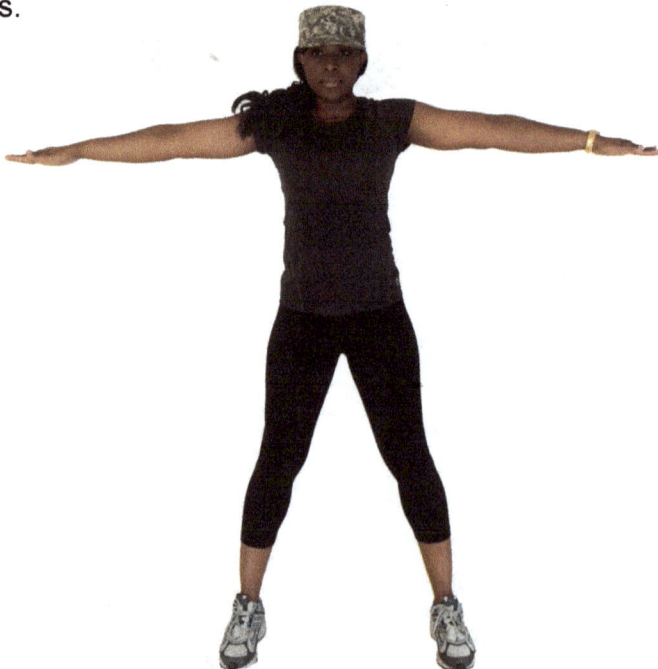

WIND MILLS

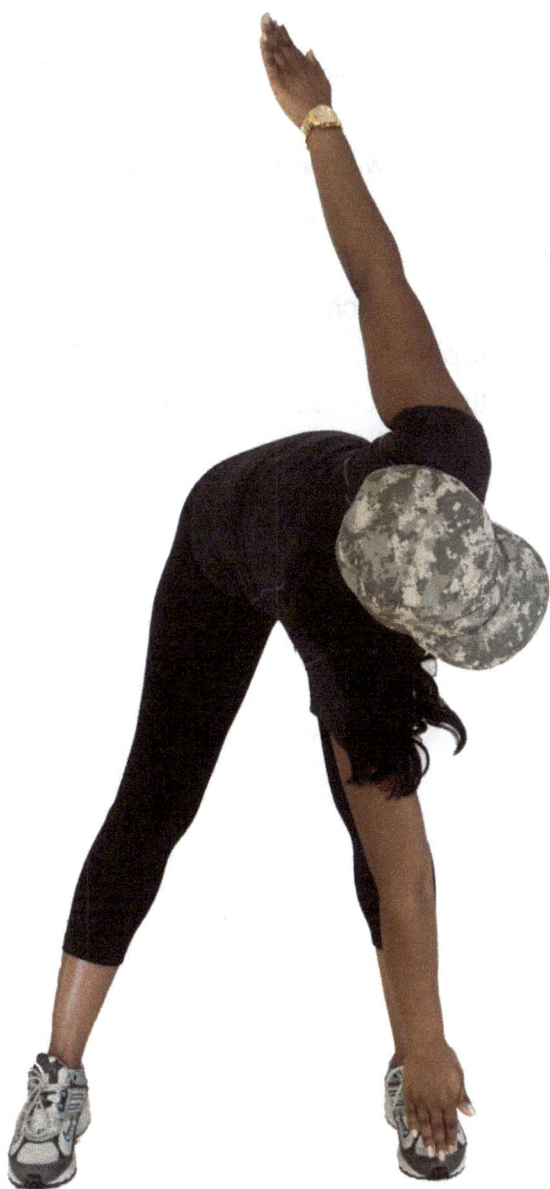

Y RAISE

Works the **upper back and shoulders.**

Lie on the floor with your face down and your arms spread straight over your head and parallel to the floor at a 30 degree angle. Your arms are forming the "Y." Your palms are facing each other with thumbs pointed up. To perform a repetition, raise your arms as high as you can and lower them back to the starting position.

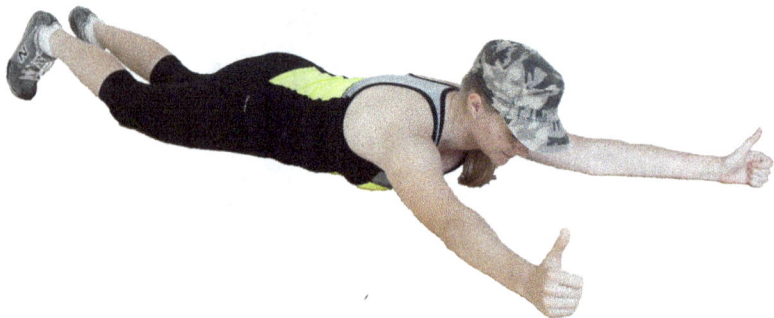

Y RAISE

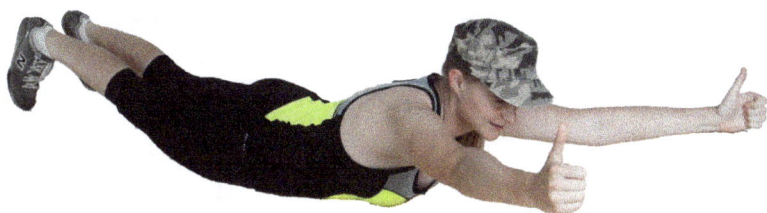

Y T I RAISES

Works **upper back and shoulders.**

You will perform the Y, T and I RAISES as separate exercises. Do 10 reps per exercise and move on to the next without resting until all three are done.

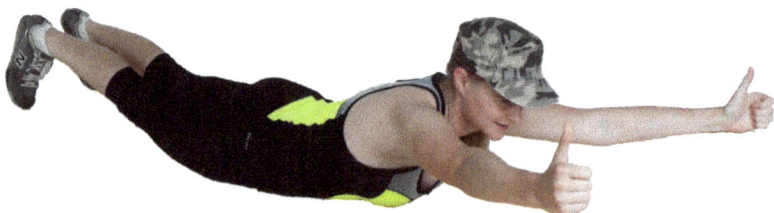

Y T I RAISES

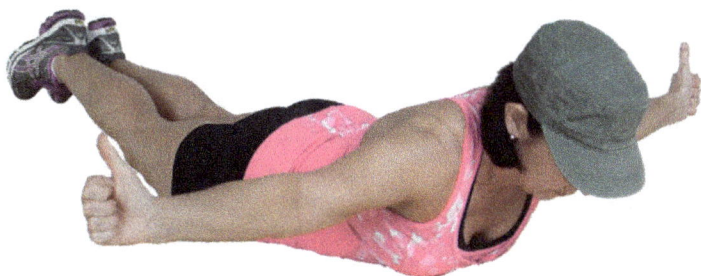

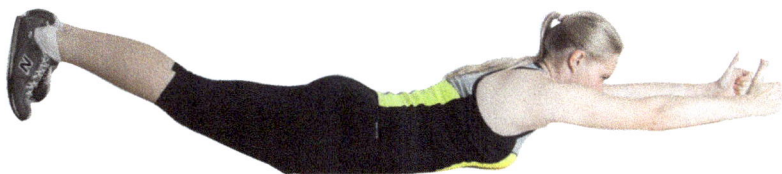

I am woman, hear me roar, in numbers too big to ignore, and I know too much to go back and pretend.
— Helen Reddy

PART C

SWISS
BALL
EXERCISES

SWISS BALL AB ROLLS

Works your **abs and other core muscles.**

Kneel down in front of the Swiss ball and place your forearms and fists on the ball. Hold your abs contracted and your back straight but with a natural spine curvature. Roll forward gradually until you feel your abs completely engaged and then back to the starting position.

Stay in touch with your body. If you notice your back is overly burdened, only go forward as far as you can without hurting yourself. You will swivel at your hips as you maintain your upper body rigid. Your arms and abdominals will be doing most of the work for this exercise.

Perform 5 - 15 repetitions of 1 to 3 sets.

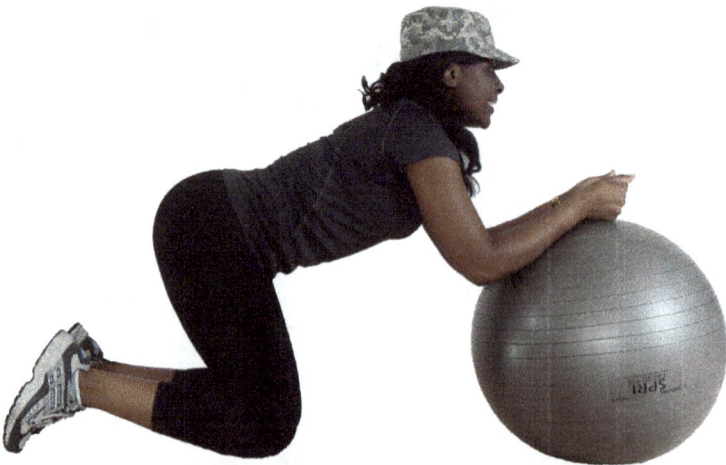

SWISS BALL AB ROLLS

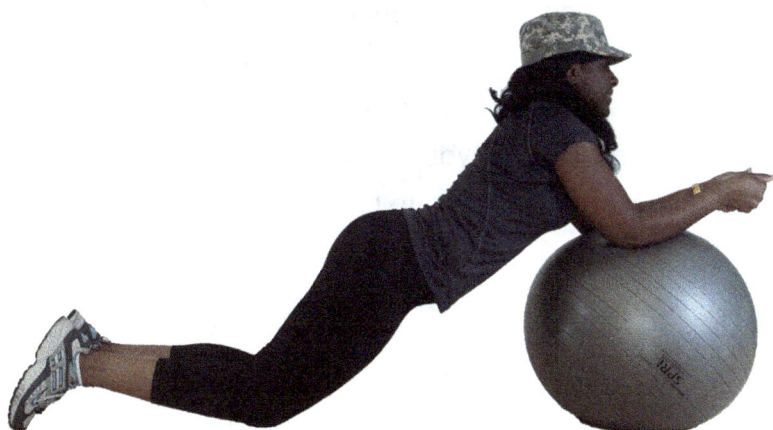

SWISS BALL DUMBBELL CHEST PRESS

Works **hips, abs, triceps, shoulders and chest**.

Take a dumbbell in each hand and place your body in such a way that your middle and upper parts of your back are firmly on the ball. Hold your body rigid and straight with your knees bent at 90 degrees. Your arms are straight up with elbows locked and your palms are facing almost completely outward. Lower the weights to the point of the sides of your chest and then back to the starting position. That is one rep.

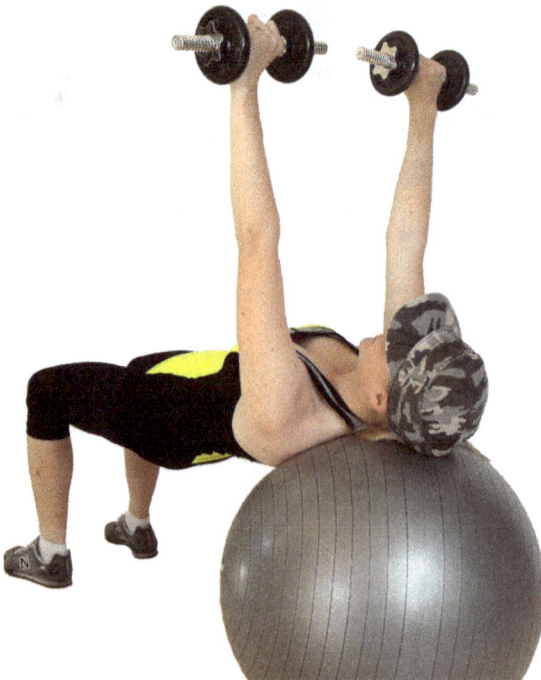

SWISS BALL DUMBBELL CHEST PRESS

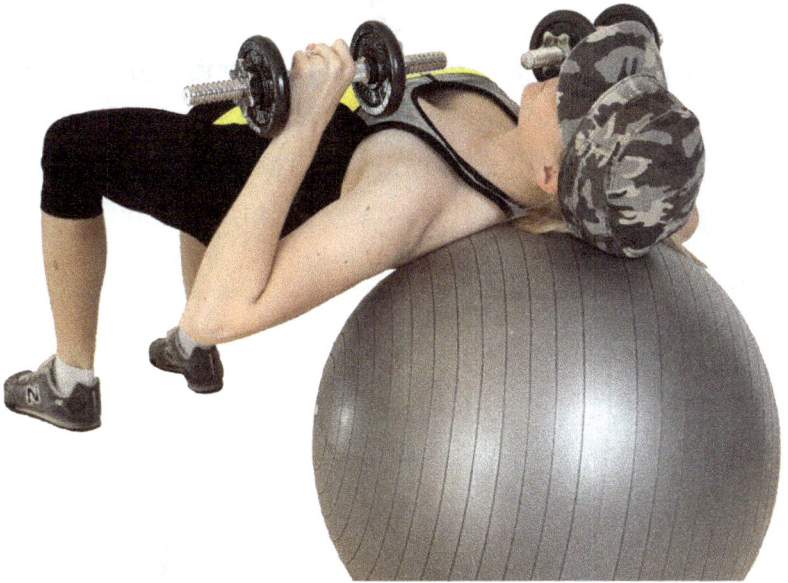

SWISS BALL HIP RAISE AND LEG CURL

Works **hamstrings, hips and butt**.

Get on your back and place your legs on a Swiss ball. Position your arms to your sides at a 90 degree angle with palms facing up. Raise your butt up to the point where your body is straight while keeping your legs on the Swiss ball and then pull the ball with your heels rolling it as close to your butt as you can. Then roll the ball back to the position with your body straight, then lower your butt back to the floor. That is one rep.

You can also modify this exercise by simply raising and lowering your butt without pulling the ball with your heels toward you.

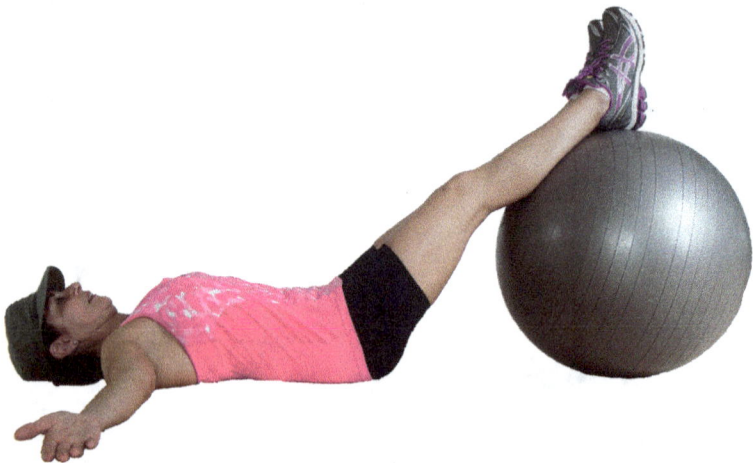

SWISS BALL HIP RAISE AND LEG CURL

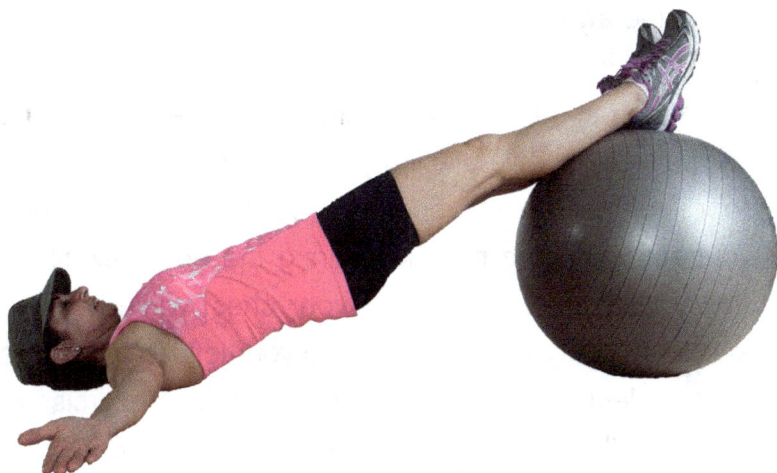

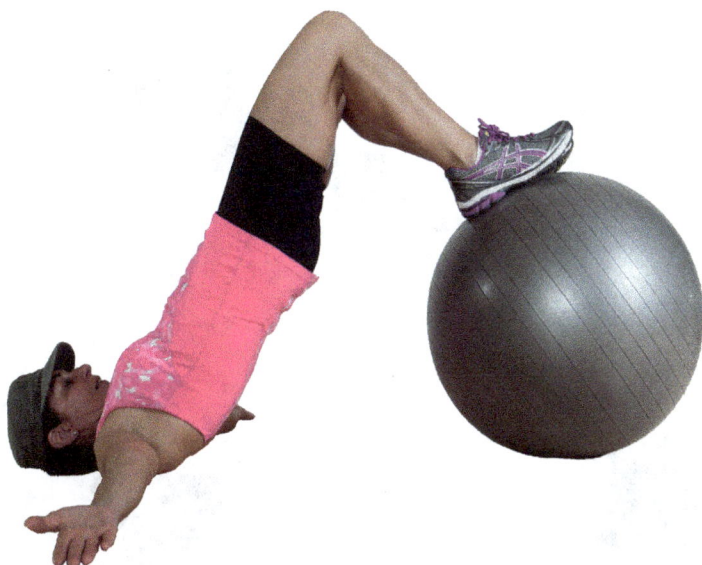

SWISS BALL MOUNTAIN CLIMBERS

Works the **entire core**.

Get in the pushup position with your arms extended and elbows locked while placing your hands on a Swiss ball. Your feet are on the floor and your body is straight. Contract your core muscles during the entire exercise. Slowly lift your right knee to your chest while keeping your body straight. Then switch to your left leg. Alternate between legs for 30 seconds. If you find this exercise to be too challenging, switch to the floor or use a bench for your hands without the Swiss ball.

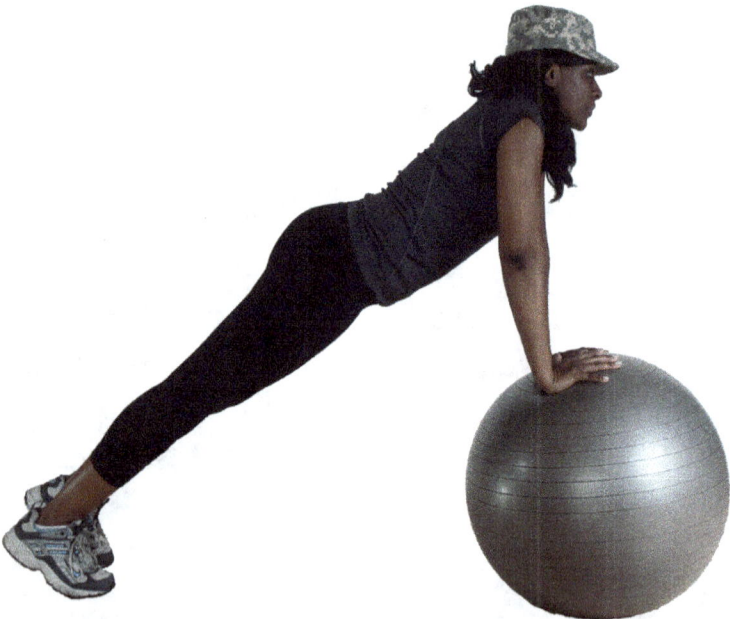

SWISS BALL MOUNTAIN CLIMBERS

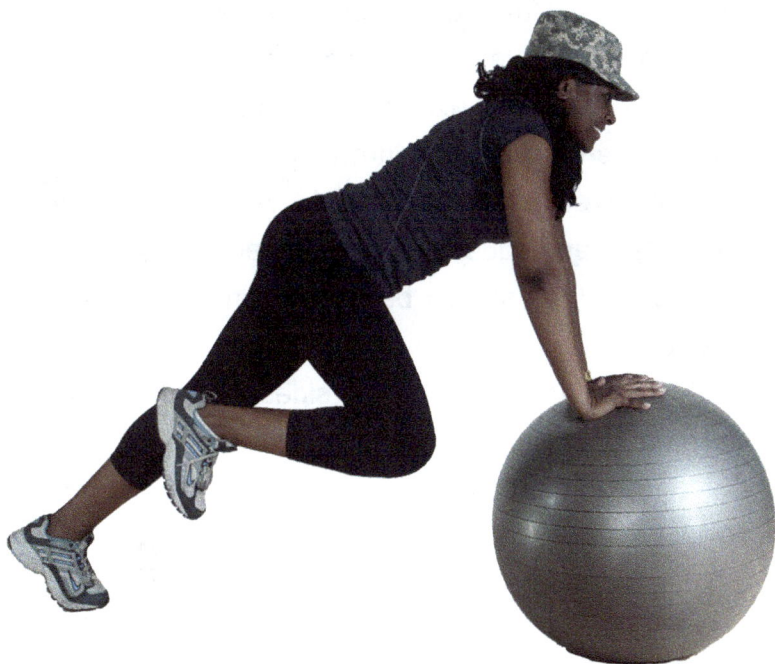

SWISS BALL RAISE

Works the **upper back and improves posture**.

Lie on the ball with your stomach on the ball; keep your back straight and your chest extended off the ball. Hang your arms down and extended with palms facing back. With elbows bent, lift your arms up as high as you can as if you were lifting dumbbells while keeping your elbows bent and squeeze the shoulder blades together. Your upper arms should be at the same level as your upper body. While maintaining your elbow position, turn your forearms up and out to the sides. Pause briefly and then take it back to the starting position. If this is too easy for you, use dumbbells.

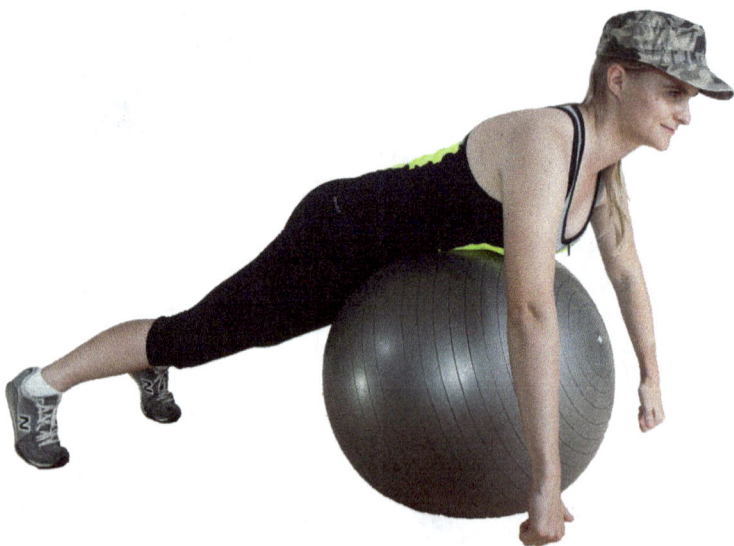

SWISS BALL RAISE

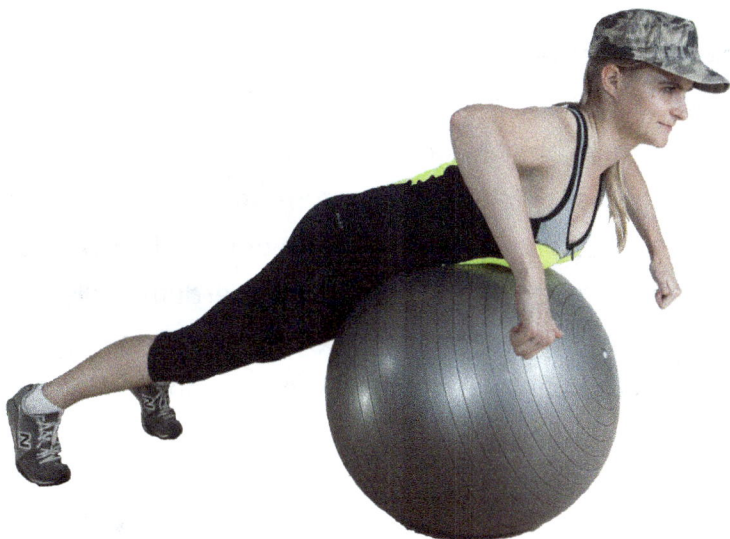

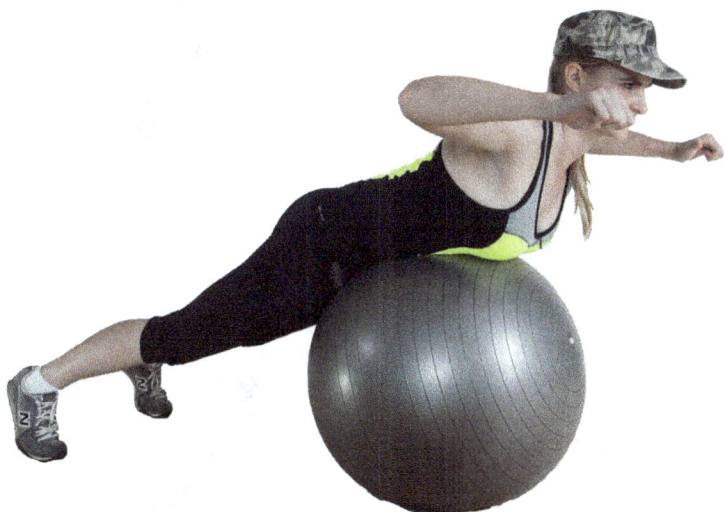

SWISS BALL TRICEPS EXTENSION

Works your **core and triceps**.

Take a dumbbell in each hand and lie with your back on a Swiss ball with your mid and upper back on the ball. Your feet are on the floor with your legs at a 90 degree angle and your body straight from knees to shoulders. With palms facing inward, hold the dumbbells over your head with straight arms up. Lower the dumbbells until they are behind your head with elbows bent and pointed up. Pause briefly and then raise the dumbbells back to the starting position.

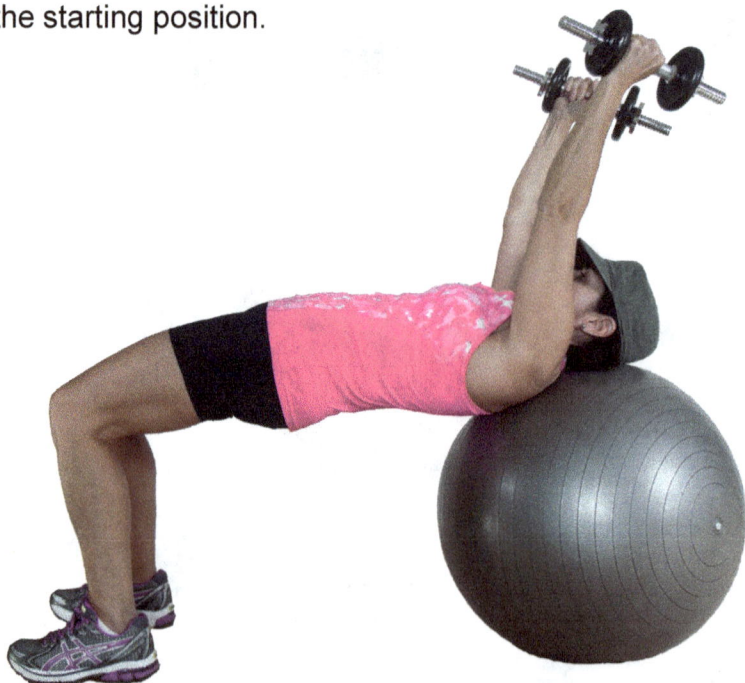

SWISS BALL TRICEPS EXTENSION

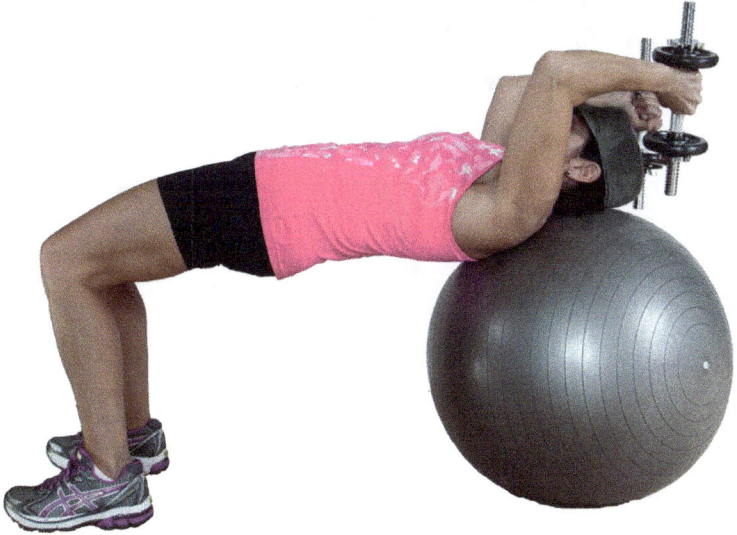

A woman is like a tea bag - you can't tell how strong she is until you put her in hot water.

— Eleanor Roosevelt

PART D

DUMBBELL EXERCISES

DUMBBELL CHEST PRESS

Works the **glutes, abs, chest and triceps**.

Lie on your back on a flat bench while holding a dumbbell in your right hand and your left hand placed on your abs. Extend your right arm straight up with the dumbbell and lower it back down to your chest while your palm is facing out and turned slightly inward. Pause briefly and then repeat. Do 10 repetitions and then switch arms and repeat.

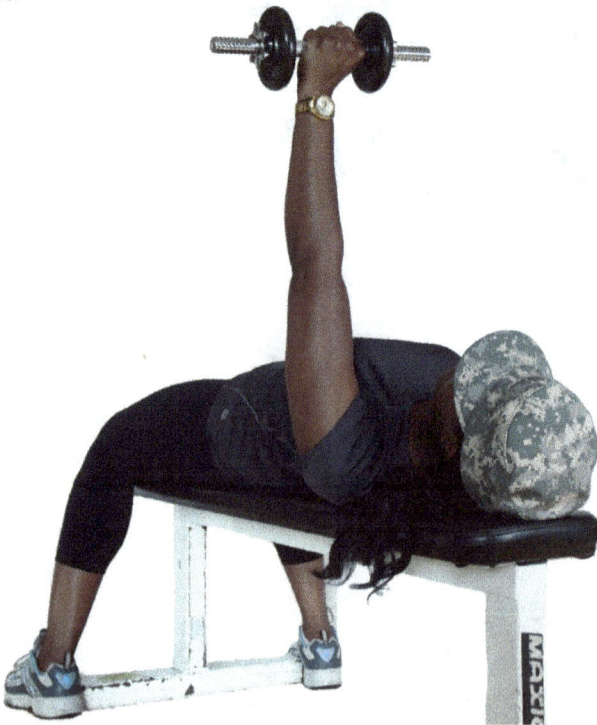

DUMBBELL CHEST PRESS

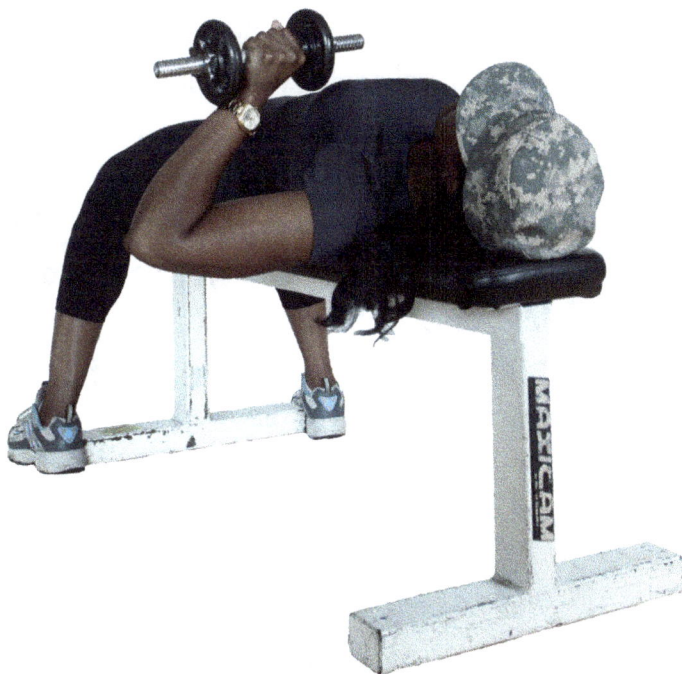

DUMBBELL CURL WITH SPLIT STANCE

Works **biceps, hip and core muscles**.

With dumbbell in each hand and in the standing position, place your right foot on an elevated surface such as a bench or step at about knee high level. Allow your dumbbells to hang at your sides with extended arms and palms facing forward. Perform a biceps curl by lifting the dumbbells while your upper arms remain stationary. You simply bend at the elbows to perform the biceps curl. Pause briefly and then gradually lower the dumbbells to the starting position.

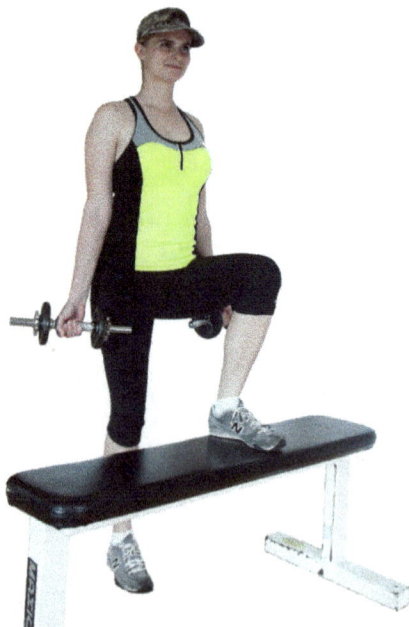

DUMBBELL CURL WITH SPLIT STANCE

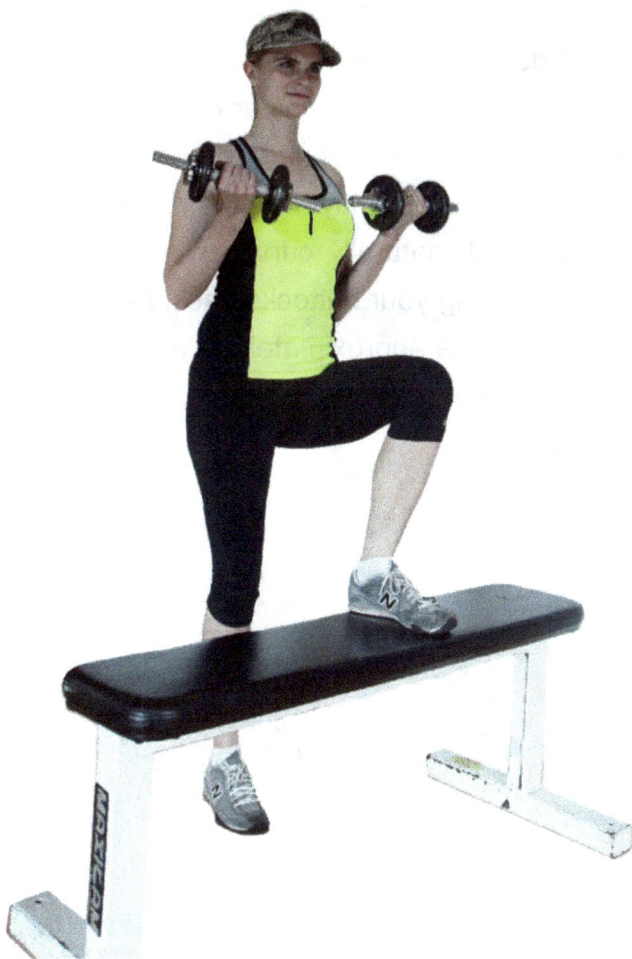

DUMBBELL GOBLET SQUAT

Works **hips and thighs**.

Take one dumbbell, pick it up and hold it with two hands in a vertical position next to your chest. Make sure you use a weight that is appropriate for you. You are standing with your feet slightly wider than shoulder width. Keep your back naturally curved without bending forward or extending your buttocks back, bend your knees until your legs are approximately at a 90 degree angle. Pause briefly and return to the starting position. That is one rep.

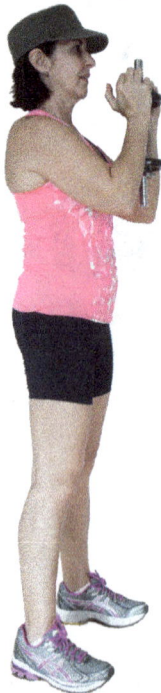

DUMBBELL GOBLET SQUAT

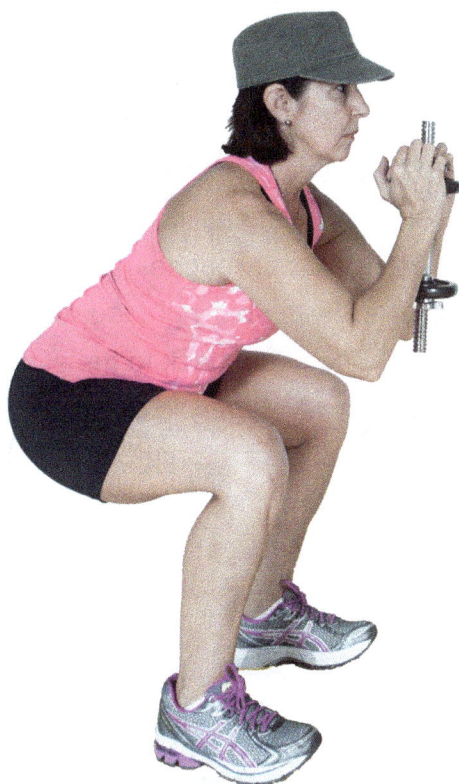

DUMBBELL LUNGE AND ROTATION

Works **hips, thighs and abs**.

Take a dumbbell and hold it with both hands chest high by holding each end. You are in the standing position with feet approximately shoulder width apart. Lunge forward with your right leg until it is at a 90 degree angle and your left knee almost reaches the floor. While you are lunging forward with your right leg, twist your upper body to the right. Then step back to the starting position with feet shoulder width apart. You have two options. You can alternate between the right and left leg for each rep or you can perform several reps with the right leg only and then switch to the left and do the same.

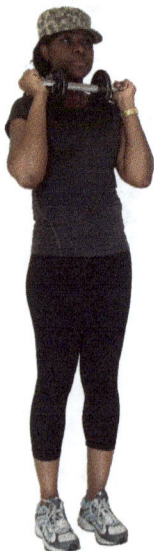

DUMBBELL LUNGE AND ROTATION

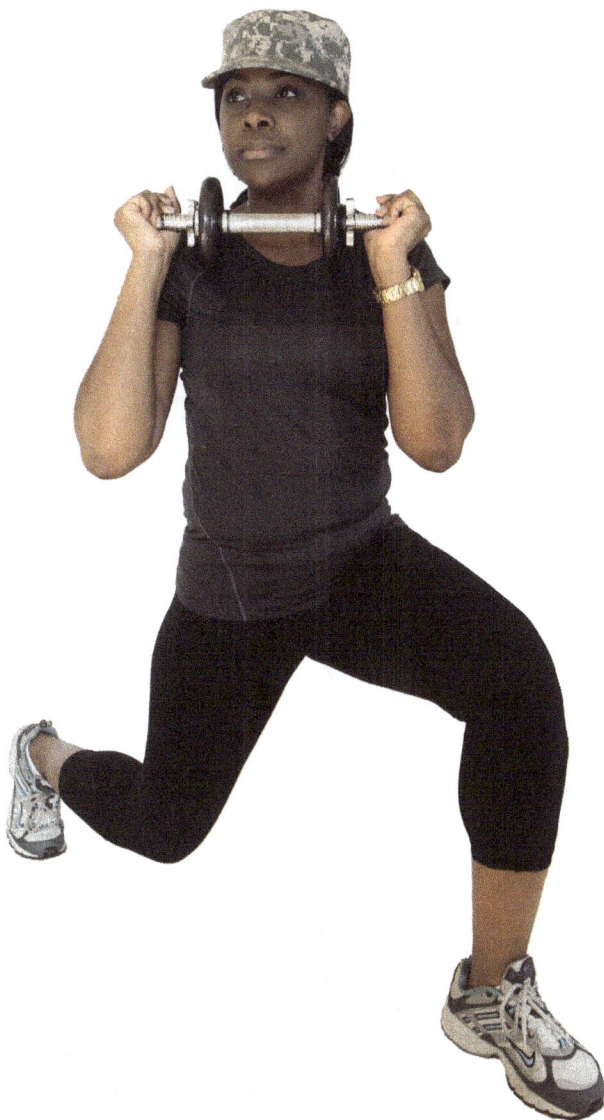

DUMBBELL PUSH PRESS

Works **triceps, hips, shoulders and thighs**.

Take a dumbbell in each hand and hold them neck high close to your shoulders while standing with your feet shoulder width apart. Go down in the lower squat position to the point where your knees are at a 90 degree angle. Then, while bringing your body back up, lift the dumbbells to the point where your arms are straight and lower the dumbbells back to the start position. That is one rep.

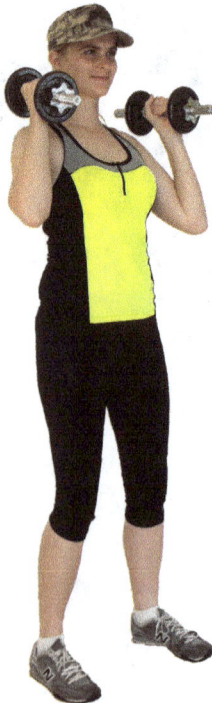

DUMBBELL PUSH PRESS

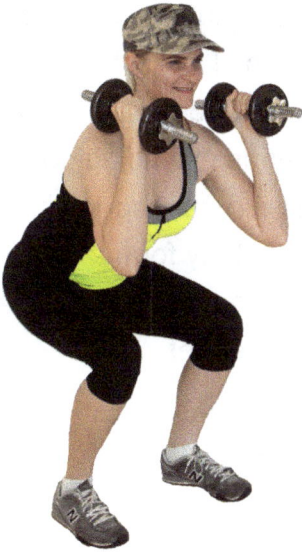

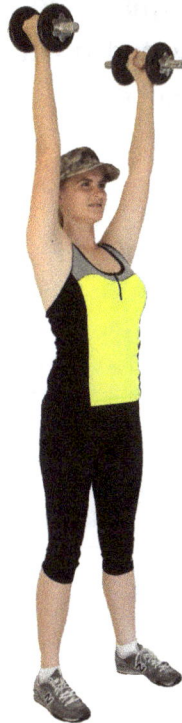

DUMBBELL REAR LATERAL RAISE

Works **shoulders and upper back**.

Stand with your feet shoulder width apart with your knees slightly bent and a dumbbell in each hand. Bend at your hips and lower your upper body until it is almost parallel to the floor with your arms extending downward and palms facing out. That is the starting position. Lift your arms out to your sides until they form a "T." Pause briefly and gradually lower them back to the starting position. Perform 10 to 20 reps per set.

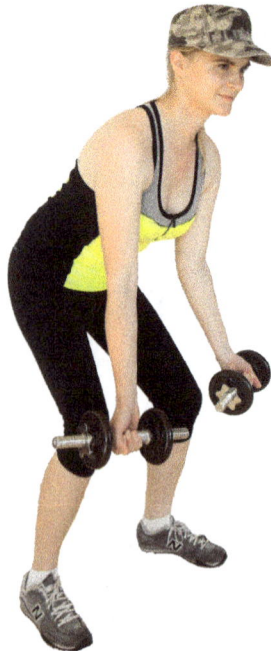

DUMBBELL REAR LATERAL RAISE

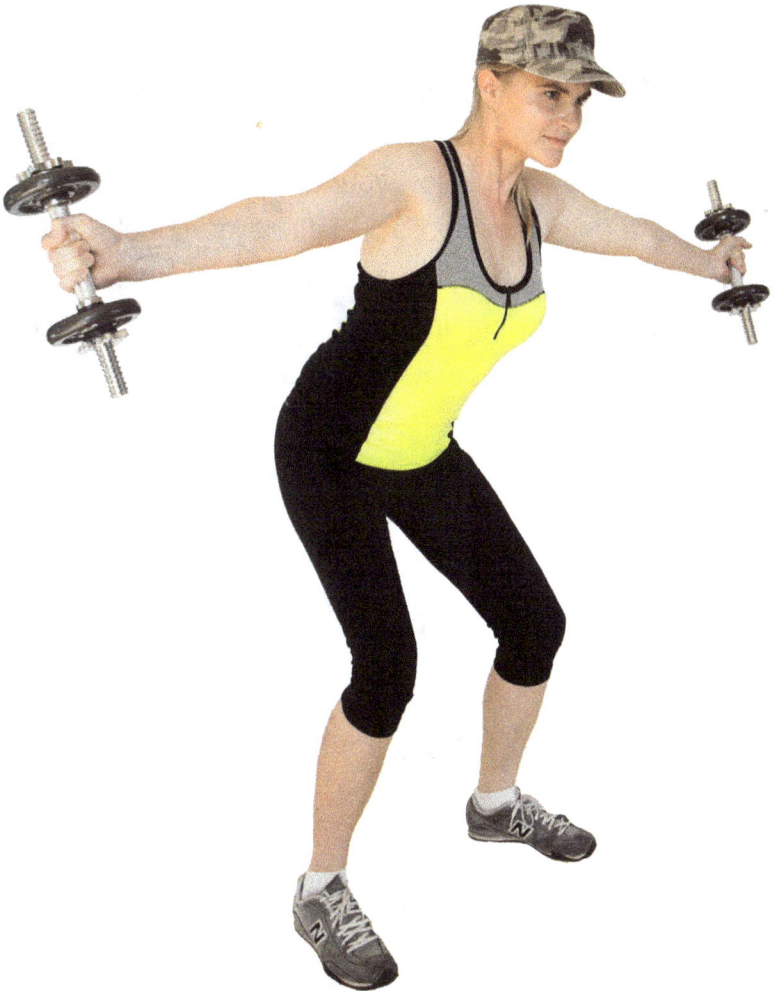

DUMBBELL ROW

Works your **biceps and back**.

With a dumbbell in each hand, stand with your knees bent slightly to stabilize the lower back and feet spread shoulder width apart. Allow your arms to extend hanging down with palms facing back. Lift the dumbbells to the point where your upper arms are parallel to the floor and your palms are still facing back. Pause briefly and then lower the dumbbells back to the starting position.

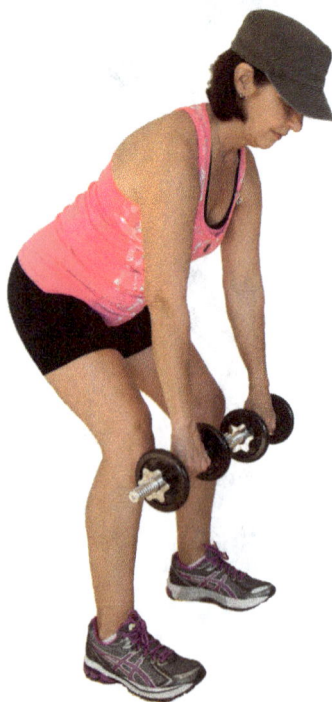

DUMBBELL ROW

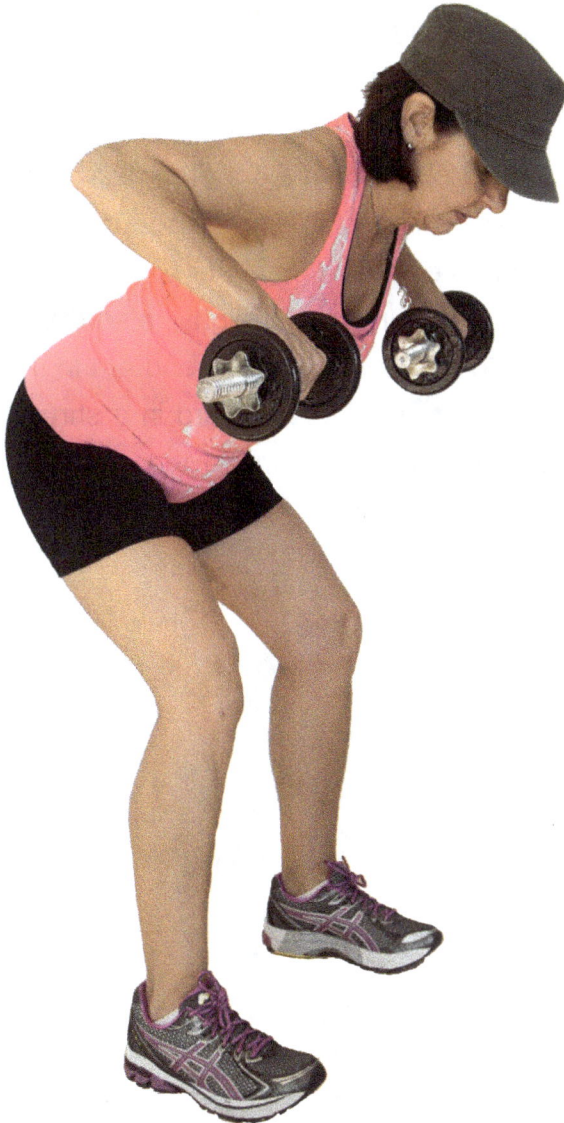

DUMBBELL SCAPTION AND SHRUG

Works the **shoulders, rotator cuff and muscle balance**. Great exercise to help **improve posture**.

In the standing position, hold a dumbbell in each hand at your sides with your feet spread about shoulder width with your arms extended and your palms facing inward. While keeping your arms straight, raise them forward until they are parallel to the floor and are in a Y formation. Move your shoulders upward in a shrugging motion and pause. Then return to the starting position. Perform 10 repetitions or more.

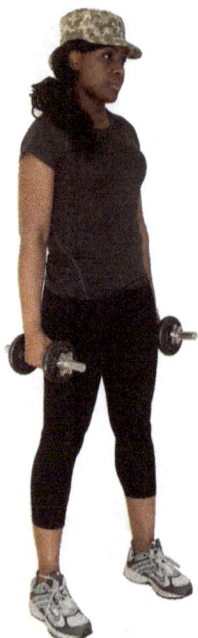

DUMBBELL SCAPTION AND SHRUG

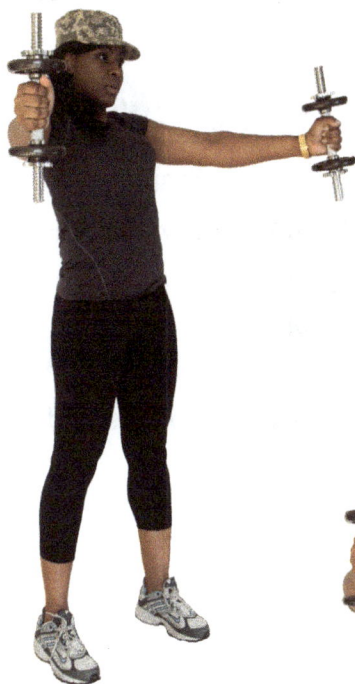

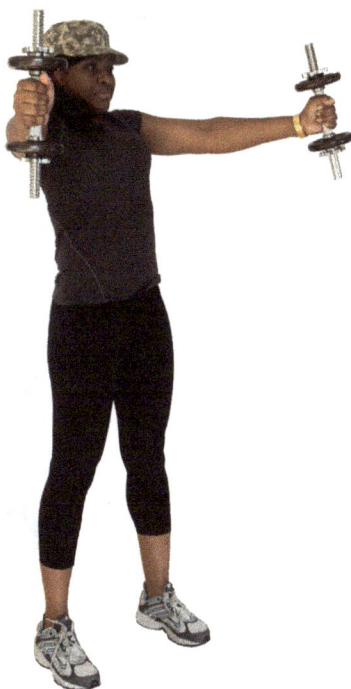

DUMBBELL STRAIGHT-LEG LIFT

Works the **hamstrings, glutes, core, muscle balance and flexibility**.

Pick up a pair of dumbbells with palms facing back and arms extended in front of your legs. Standing with your feet approx. shoulder-width apart and your knees bent slightly, raise your right leg off the floor and extend it back while lowering your upper body where it is parallel to the floor. Pause briefly, then bring your body back to the starting position by squeezing your glutes and thrusting your hips forward.

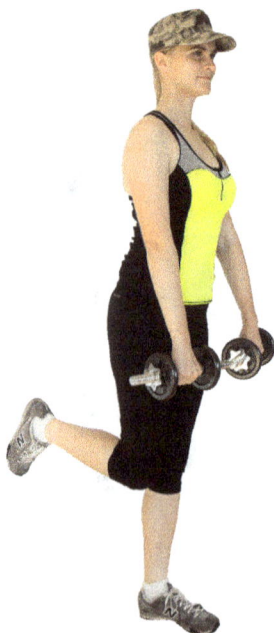

DUMBBELL STRAIGHT-LEG LIFT

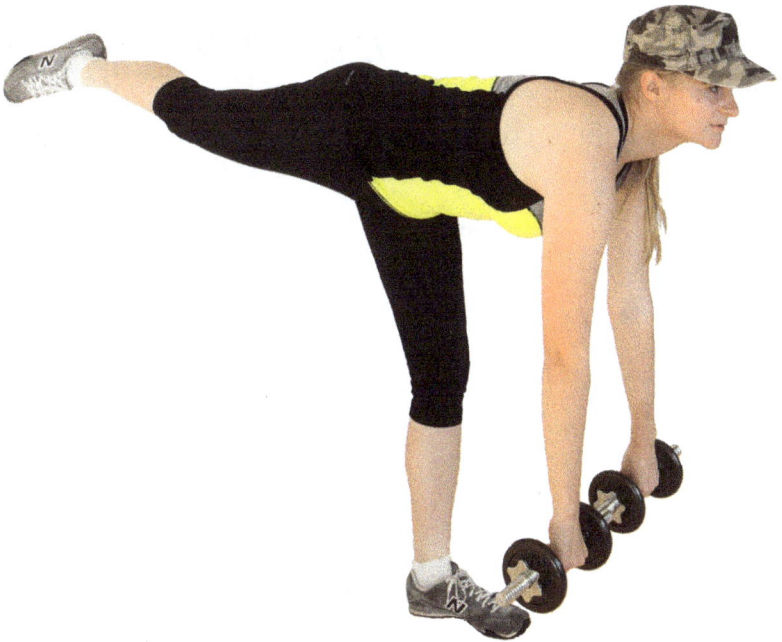

OFFSET DUMBBELL LUNGE

Works the **quads, core and balance**.

Your right arm is bent while holding a dumbbell next to your neck. Lunge forward with your right leg until your leg is at a 90 degree angle with your left knee almost touching the floor. Push your body back up to the standing position. That is one repetition. Do 10 reps with the right leg forward and then 10 with your left leg forward.

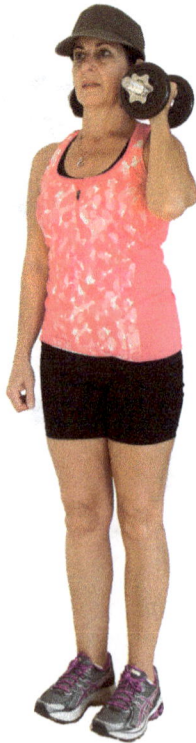

OFFSET DUMBBELL LUNGE

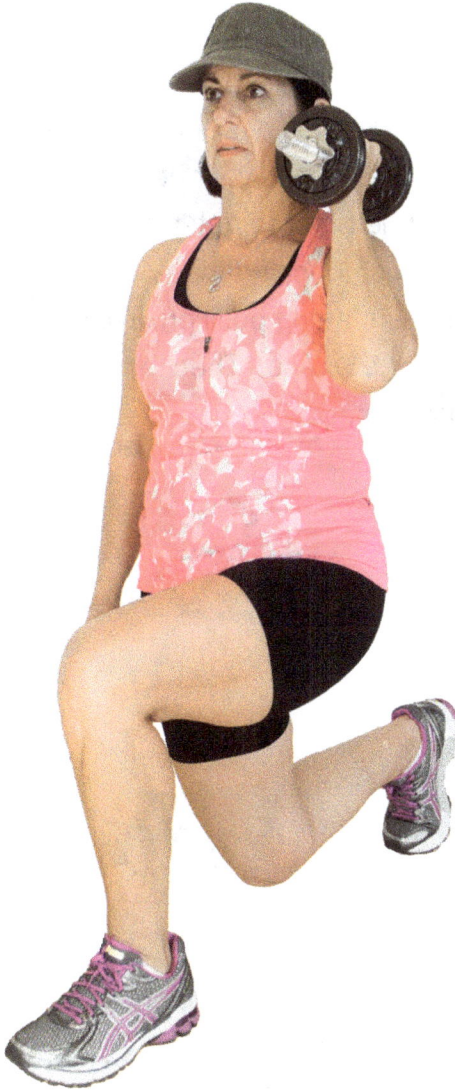

OFFSET REVERSE DUMBBELL LUNGE

Works **hips, thighs and abs**.

You are in the standing position with a dumbbell in your right hand, raised next to your head with arm bent. Step back with your left foot to get into a lunge position with your knee almost touching the floor then bring your left foot back to the starting position. That is one repetition. Perform 30 to 50 reps. Then alternate position and perform another set.

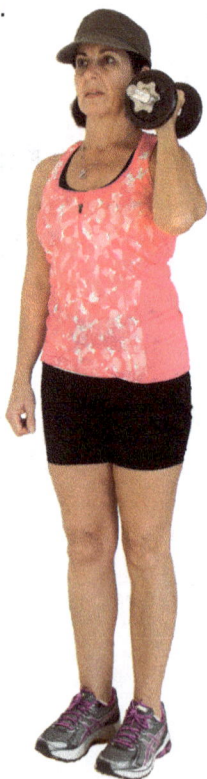

OFFSET REVERSE DUMBBELL LUNGE

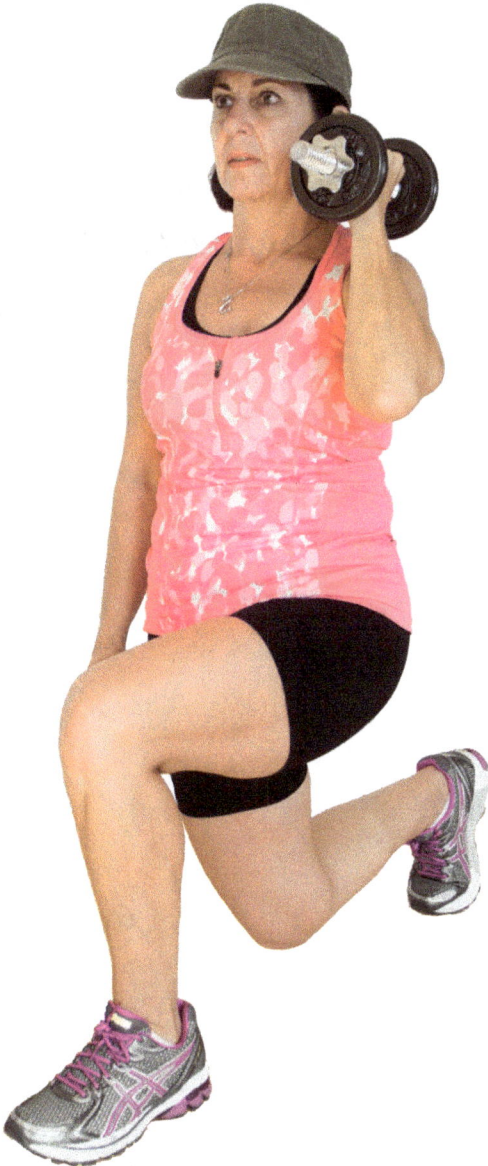

The practice of putting women on pedestals began to die out when it was discovered that they could give orders better from there.

— *Betty Grable*

PART E

RESISTANCE
BAND
EXERCISES

BICEPS CURLS

Works the **biceps.**

Grab each handle with your left and right hand. Your feet are shoulder width apart and you are standing firmly on the band with the band in the center of your shoes. Bend your knees slightly to stabilize your lower back with your palms facing out and your arms extended down. Pull the band up to your shoulder joint and resist it going down.

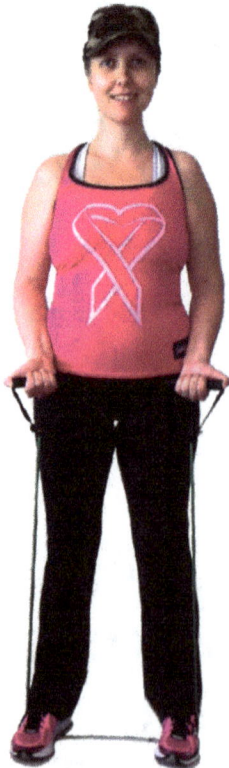

Part E - Resistance Band Exercises

BICEPS CURLS

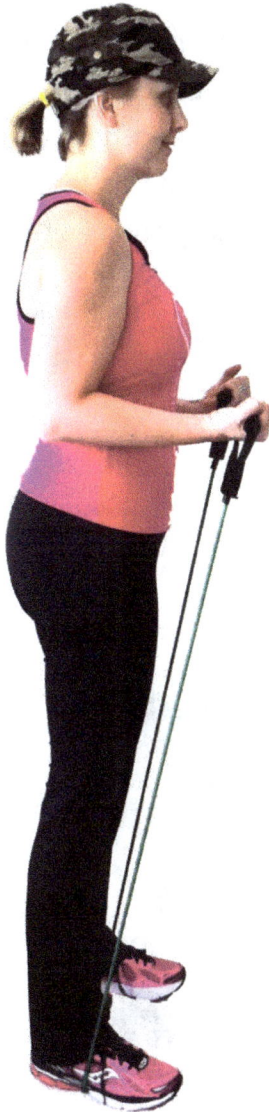

FRONT RAISE

Works the **shoulders and front deltoids.**

Grab each handle with your left and right hand. Your left foot is forward and on the band. Extend your arms forward, lock your elbows and hold your wrists straight with palms facing down. Pull the band upward to where the arms are parallel to the ground and resist it going back down.

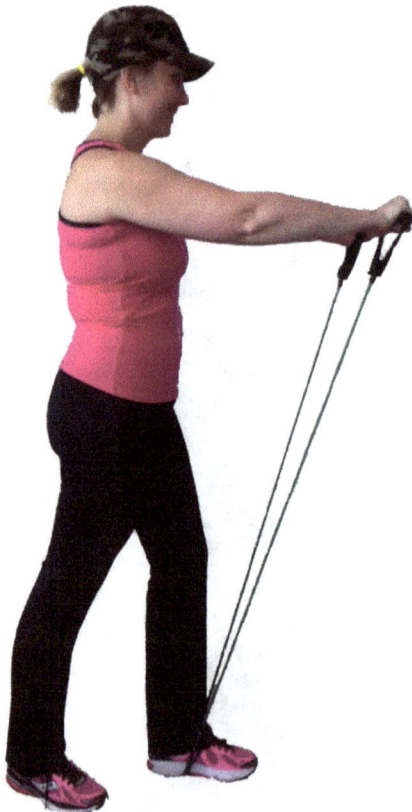

FRONT RAISE

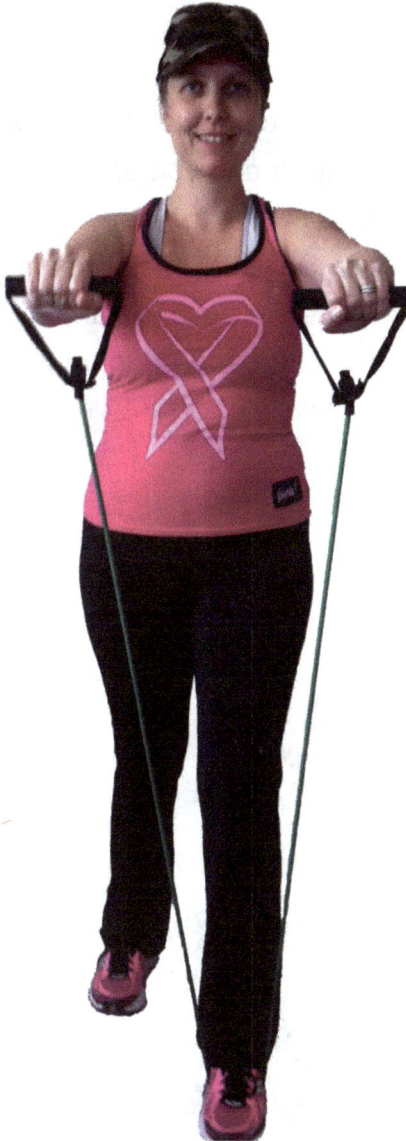

REVERSE CURLS

Works the **biceps and forearms.**

Grab each handle with your left and right hand. Your feet are shoulder width apart and you are standing firmly on the band with the band in the center of your shoes. Maintain a slight bend in your knees to stabilize the lower back. Your palms are facing back and your arms are extended down. Pull the band up to your shoulder joint and resist it going down.

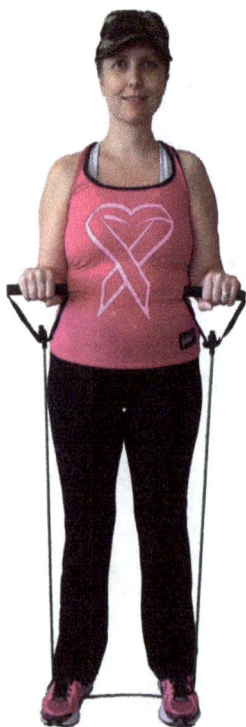

REVERSE CURLS

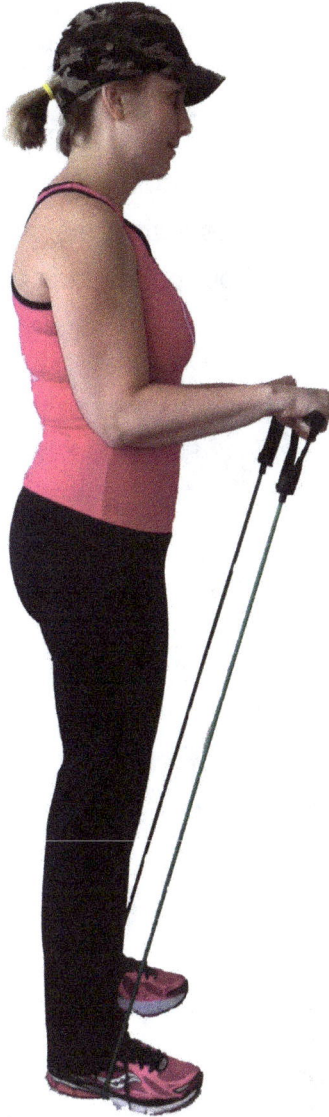

SIDE LATERAL RAISE

Works the **shoulders, core muscles and arms.**

Grab each handle with your left and right hand. Your left foot is forward and on the band. Extend your arms out to the sides, lock your elbows with arms straight and hold your wrists straight with your palms facing down. Pull the band up until the arms are parallel to the ground and resist it going back down.

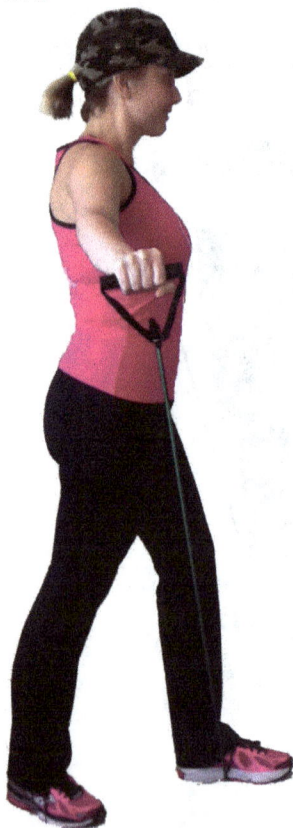

SIDE LATERAL RAISE

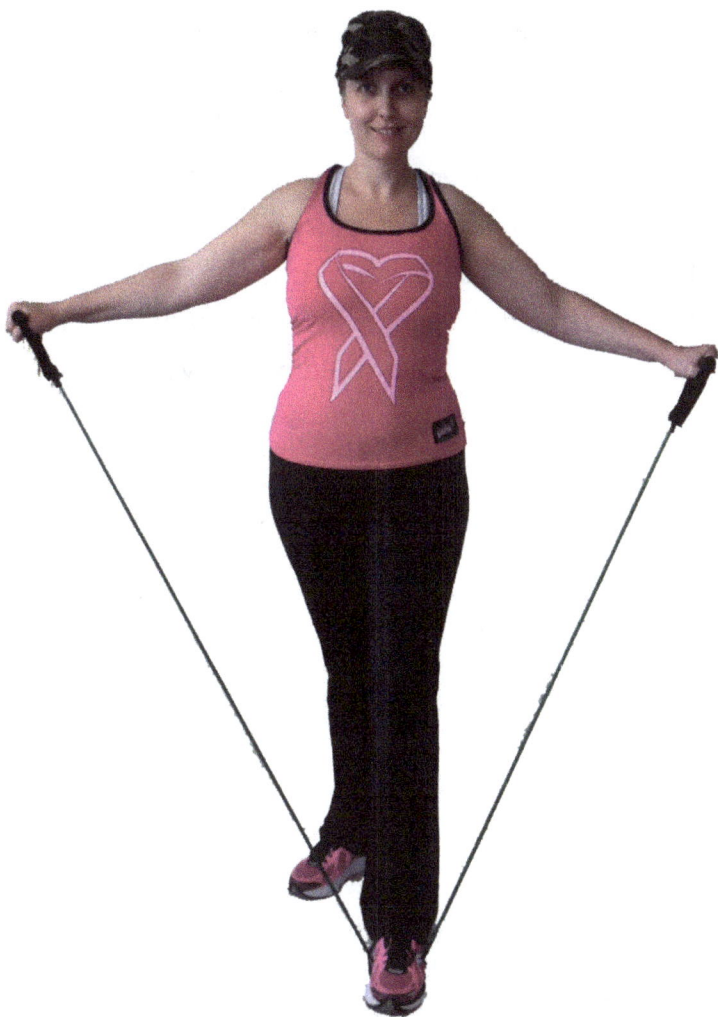

TRICEPS PUSH

Works the **triceps**.

Take the band in your right hand and place the other end on the ground in front of your right foot. Place your right foot six to eight inches into the band and firmly onto to the band with the ball of your foot so that it doesn't slip. Now step forward with your left foot while keeping your right foot on the band. Take your right hand with the band handle and bring it up behind your head. The starting position is with the hand lowered behind your head. Push up on the band until the arm is completely extended. That's one rep. Switch hands and feet and do the same thing with the left side of your body.

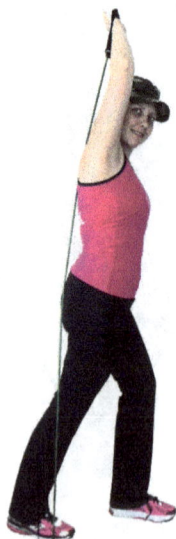

TRICEPS PUSH

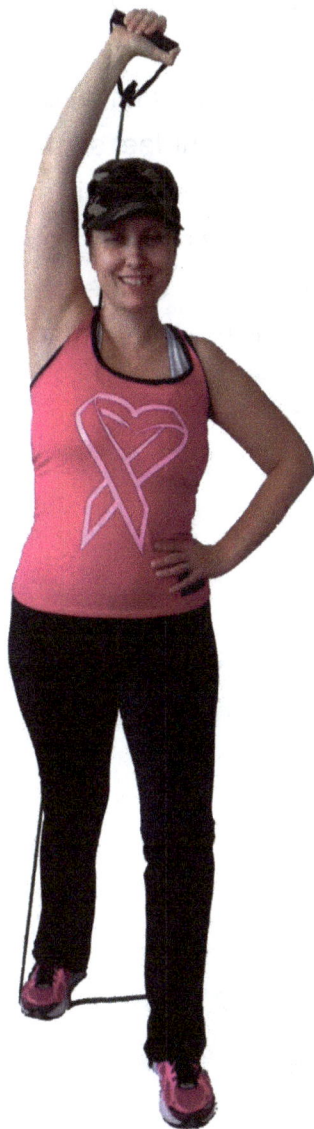

UPRIGHT ROW

Works the **lats, traps and arms.**

Grab each handle with your left and right hand. Place two feet on the band with your feet shoulder width apart. With both wrists hanging down, pull the band up to your shoulder joint while maintaining your wrists in the down position and then back to the starting position while resisting it going down.

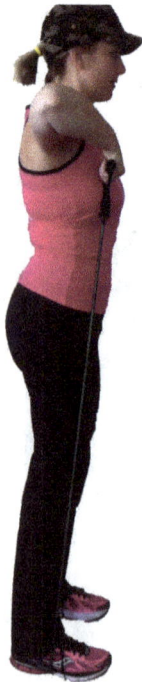

UPRIGHT ROW

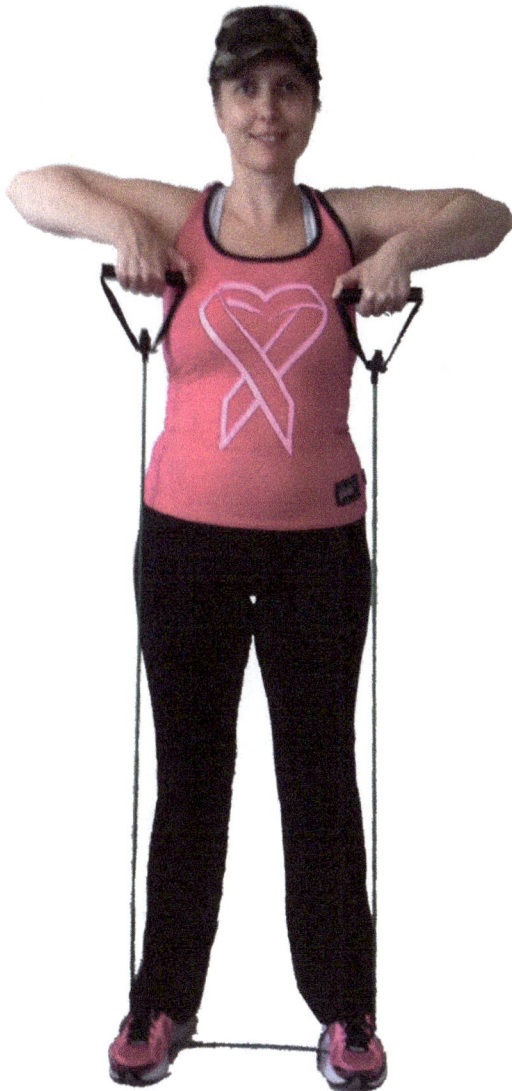

I would rather trust a woman's instinct than a man's reason.
— Stanley Baldwin

PART F

15 MINUTE WORKOUTS

READ THIS FIRST
15 MINUTE WORKOUTS

For those who have little time and would like to maximize the health and fitness benefit, a 15 minute workout designed as circuit training is a great way to get your cardio as well as complete body strength training. Each of the 15 minute workouts have seven exercises. You will perform each of the seven exercise for 60 seconds, then take a 60 second break and perform all seven again, 60 seconds each. Pace yourself so that you can complete the entire 15 minutes. If an exercise should become too fatiguing for you, simply modify it and slow the pace to the point where you still continue. If, for some reason, you cannot perform an exercise, select a suitable alternative that you can perform. Do not be discouraged if you find it hard to maintain and complete the entire 15 minutes. Remember your primary purpose for exercising and that is your health. If you are feeling fatigued during the workout you are making progress. You must feel some fatigue to make progress. One of my favorite quotes of which I am the author of during my beach boot camp classes is this:

"You must meet my friend Fatigue before you can meet my friend Progress. Fatigue is the gatekeeper to Progress."

15 MINUTE WORKOUT
GUIDELINES

- Perform each exercise for 60 seconds.
- Perform the same 7 exercises, 60 seconds each.
- Take a 60 second break after cycling through the 7 exercises.
- Pace yourself so you can complete the entire cycles.
- Modify an exercise, if necessary, to keep going.
- Slow your pace, if necessary, to keep going.
- Form is not as important as movement, unless you may hurt yourself by compromising form.
- Listen to your body.
- You may feel soreness up to 3 days after a 15 minute workout.
- You can workout every day with these 15 minute workouts. You may simply need to go easy on a body part.
- You can warm up by going for a run, jogging in place, performing pushups, crunches or some other exercise.
- You can also make your warm up a part of your 15 minute workout by pacing yourself a little slower with the first couple of exercises and then picking up the pace.

WORKOUT A

1. Burpees
2. T Pushup
3. High Kick
4. Incline Pushup
5. High Step
6. Hip Raise
7. Crunches

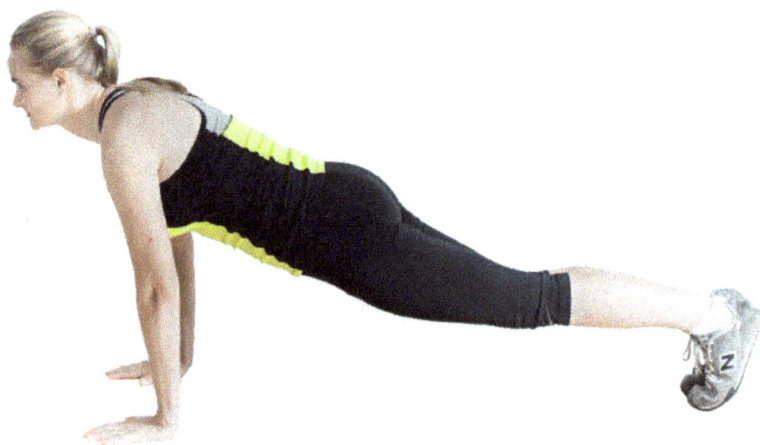

WORKOUT B

1. Jumping Jacks
2. Dumbbell Push Press
3. Squats
4. Dumbbell Scaption and Shrug
5. Stationary Lunges
6. Dumbbell Row
7. Swiss Ball Mountain Climbers

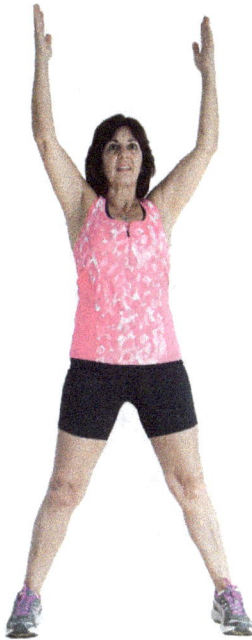

WORKOUT C

1. Dumbbell Lunge and Rotation
2. Spiderman Pushup
3. Dumbbell Goblet Squat
4. Side Kick and Punch
5. Crunches
6. T Pushup
7. Dumbbell Curl and Split

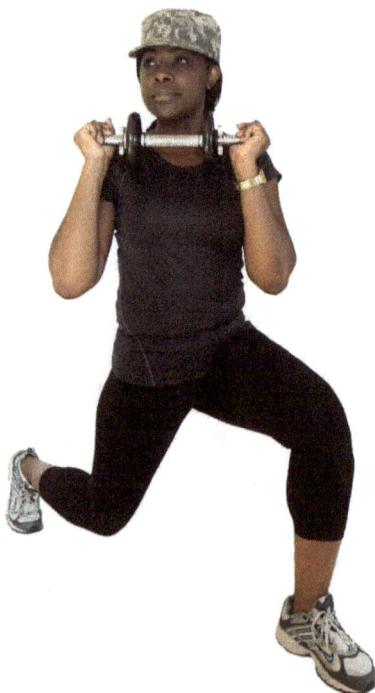

WORKOUT D

1. Swiss Ball Raise
2. Swiss Ball Triceps Extension
3. Squats
4. Swiss Ball Dumbbell Chest Press
5. Swiss Ball Hip Raise and Leg Curl
6. Reverse Crunch
7. Swiss Ball Raise

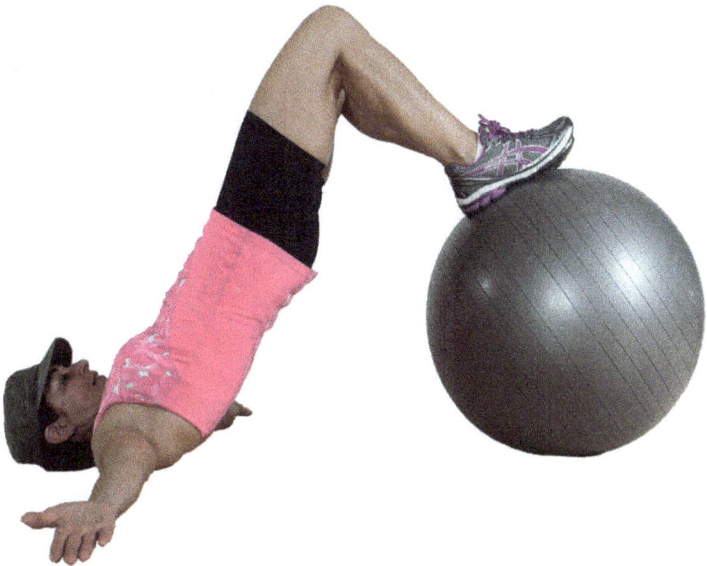

WORKOUT E

1. Mountain Climber
2. Crunches
3. Regular Pushup
4. Crunches
5. Squats
6. Crunches
7. Triceps Pushups

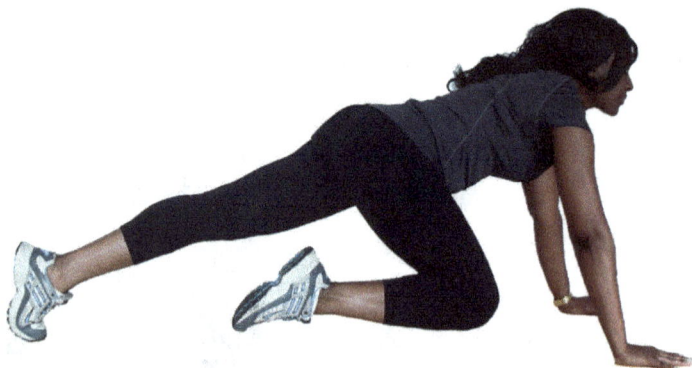

WORKOUT F

1. Dumbbell Straight-leg Lift
2. Side Plank
3. Mountain Climber
4. Dumbbell Rear Lateral Raise
5. Hip Raise
6. Regular Pushup
7. Crunches

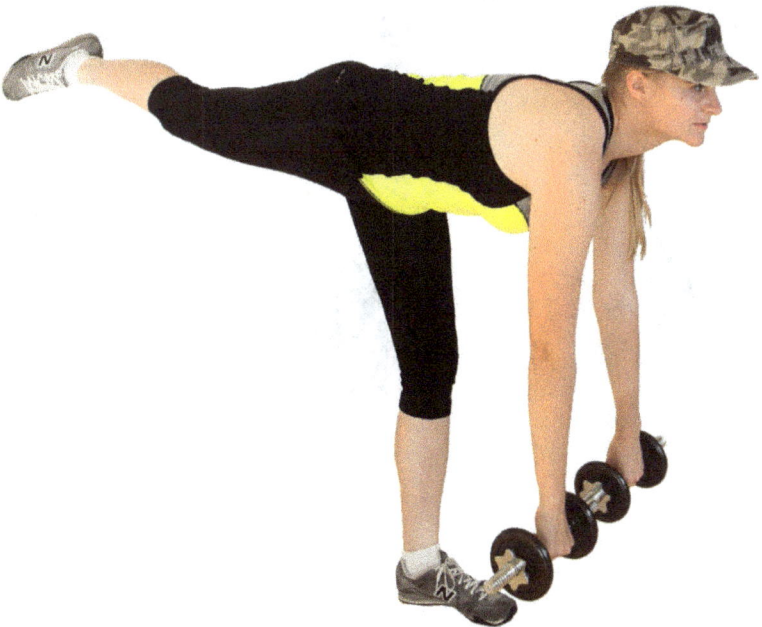

WORKOUT G

1. Regular Pushups
2. Crunches
3. Wide Pushup
4. Situps
5. Tricep Pushups
6. Flutter Kicks
7. Crunches with Legs Straight Up

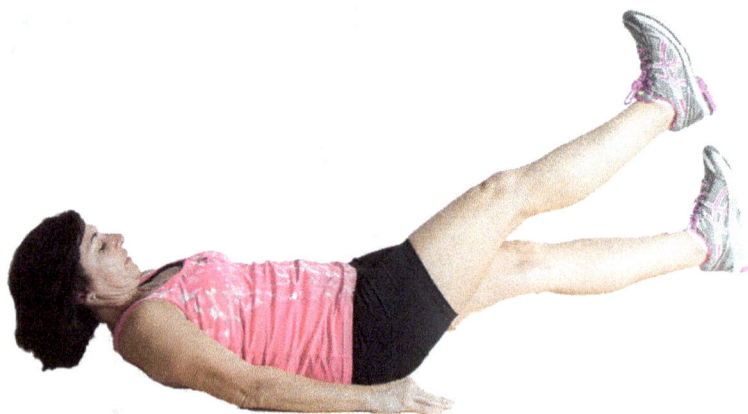

WORKOUT H

1. High Step
2. Windmills
3. Jumping Jacks
4. High Kick
5. Squats
6. High Step
7. Knee Thrust

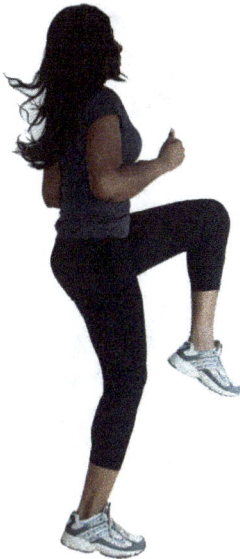

154 | Boot Camp for Women

WORKOUT I

1. Windmills
2. Squats
3. Crunches
4. Regular Pushup
5. Stationary Lunges
6. Crunches
7. Squats

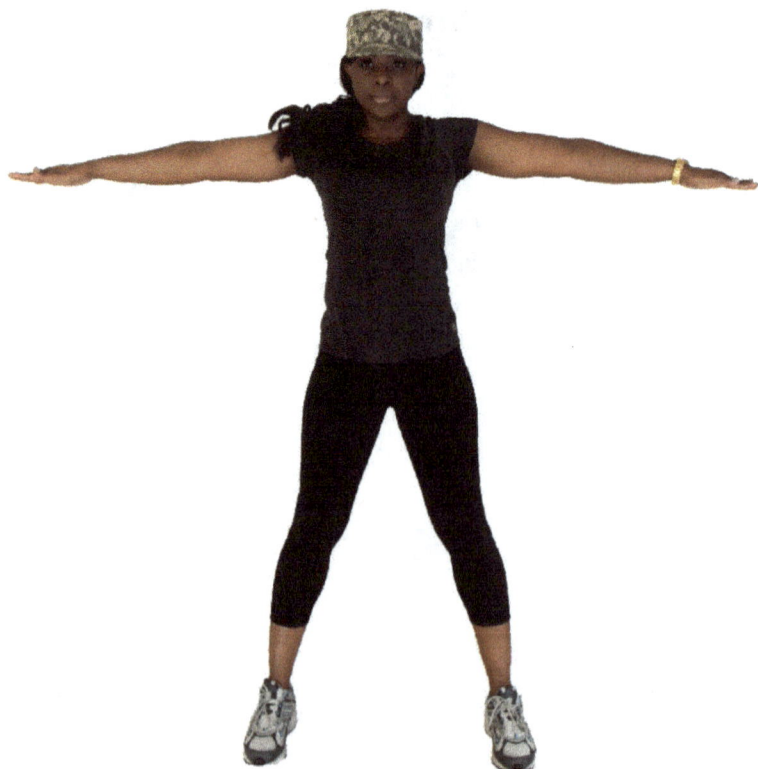

WORKOUT J

Design Your Own Workout

With the random workout you can spontaneously decide which exercises you will use for your 15 minute workout. Remember, it's seven exercises of one minute each. Then take a 60 second break and perform seven more exercises. For the random workout the second seven exercises do not have to be the same as the first seven. You can also design your 15 minute workout to focus on the body parts you want to work the most.

Exercise 1 - you choose

Exercise 2 - you choose

Exercise 3 - you choose

Exercise 4 - you choose

Exercise 5 - you choose

Exercise 6 - you choose

Exercise 7 - you choose

RPE OR RATE OF PERCEIVED EXERTION

RPE is an easy way to determine what level of exertion you are applying to your aerobic workout. In the fitness world we normally think of cardio (aerobic) and strength training as separate. Combining them will result in a new level of strength and cardiovascular conditioning. Your muscle strength training will add an important component called muscle endurance training, the ability of the muscle to continuously work while fatigued. Excellent muscle endurance is probably more important from a health standpoint than simply strong muscles. RPE is how you perceive the level of fatigue.

RPE SCALE

0	Nothing at All
1	Very Weak
2	Weak
3	Moderate
4	Somewhat Hard
5	Hard
6	
7	Very Hard
8	
9	
10	Very, Very Hard

PYRAMID WORKOUTS

Another great way to increase strength and endurance are with pyramid workouts. A pyramid workout with push-ups could, for example, be built by gradually increasing the reps for five sets and then gradually decreasing for four sets back to the starting number of reps. Pyramid workouts can be used for just about any exercise. Many times our bodies will plateau and not continue to make strength or cardio progress. The body has adapted to whatever routine we are doing. Pyramid workouts will interrupt your routine and cause your muscles to respond to strength and endurance improvements.

Example

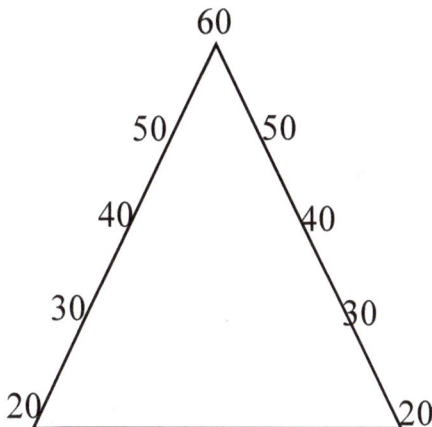

About the Author

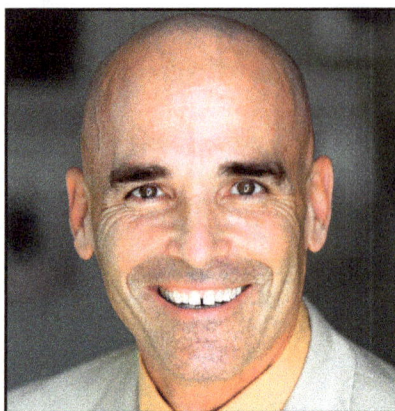

Joseph "Bob" Weinstein
Lt. Colonel, U.S. Army, Retired
www.BeachBootCamp.net
Blog: www.colonelbobsbeachbootcamp.blogspot.com/

BIO

Born in Washington, D.C., **Lt. Colonel Bob Weinstein** grew up in Virginia and spent 20 years in Berlin, Germany; he is retired from the United States Army as a Lieutenant Colonel with 30 years of service, both reserve and active duty time, and spent about half that time as a senior military instructor with the Command & General Staff College at one of the satellite locations in Germany.

He has been featured on radio and television, among others, on the History Channel and Fox Sports Net as well as in various publications such as the Washington Times, The Miami Herald and the Las Vegas Tribune.

His background is unique and diverse, including: military instructor, attorney, motivational speaker, wellness coach, certified corporate trainer, and certified personal trainer. He is fluent in German and English.

He is a popular motivational speaker at corporate events and banquets and conducts military-style workouts on Fort Lauderdale Beach utilizing strength, cardio, flexibility and agility training - both in personal training and group sessions.

Col. Weinstein has volunteered his time for homeless and run-away kids at the Covenant House and has devoted time to training youth who are members of the US Naval Sea Cadets Corps, Team Spruance, Fort Lauderdale, Florida.

He is a member of the American Council on Exercise.

Boot Camp Fitness for All Shapes and Sizes, Weight Loss - Twenty Pounds in Ten Weeks are some of his books he has authored and published. Some of his previous clients as a guest speaker include: Sony, DHL, American Express, KPMG, AOL, IBM, AARP, SmithBarney, Green Bay Packers and Humana.

Lt. Colonel Bob Weinstein
U.S. Army, Retired
954-636-5351
www.BeachBootCamp.net

Darlene Wooldridge

Darlene has been a physical therapist for over 30 years. She owns and operates Back To Health Physical Therapy in Ft. Lauderdale, Florida. Beach boot camp allows her to combine her love for the outdoors and exercise to maintain a healthy lifestyle.

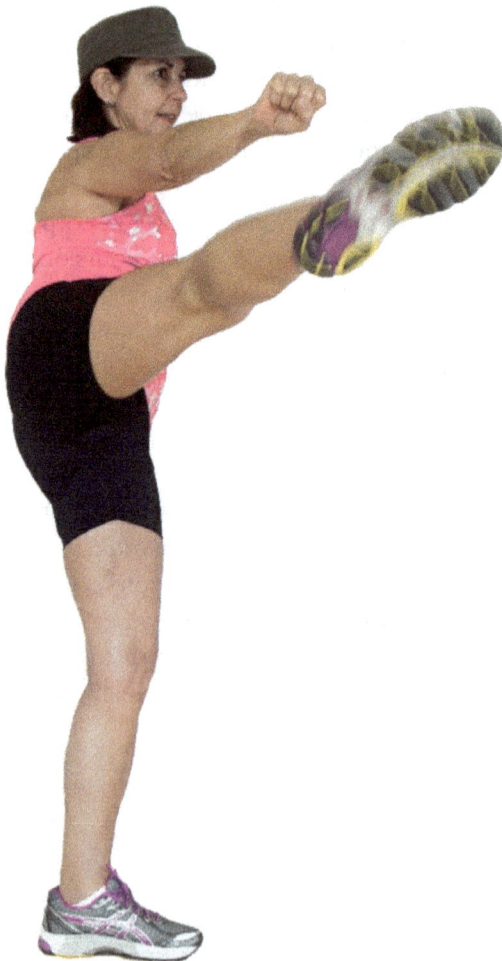

Dr. Katerina Kostioukhina with son and daughter

Dr. Kostioukhina, a graduate from the university of Miami and longstanding boot camp recruit has been pursuing her personal journey to health.

"We always tell our patients to eat healthy and exercise; but for some reason the advice doesn't seem to work. That is why I decided to try it myself. The challenge is exercising and eating healthy all while being a medical student, mother, wife and business owner. "
"The journey has not been an easy one, but the rewards in energy and well being are priceless. Eating healthy and exercising is well worth the challenge. "

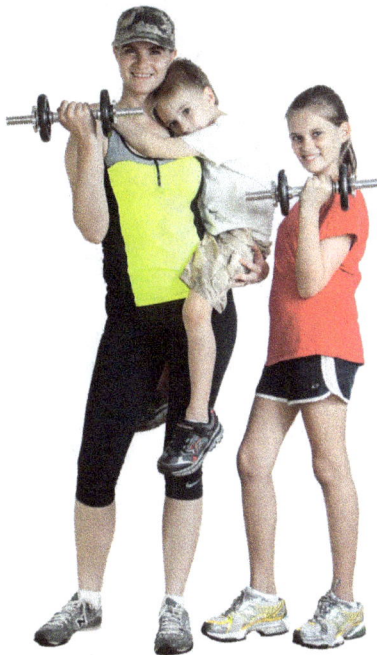

Merisia Challenger and son

Merisia is currently living in Weston, Florida. She was born in Saint Kitts and raised in New York City. She is currently working in the law enforcement field. She loves and enjoys spending time with her son. He is the joy of her life. Love, life, laughter and happiness is the motto of her life.

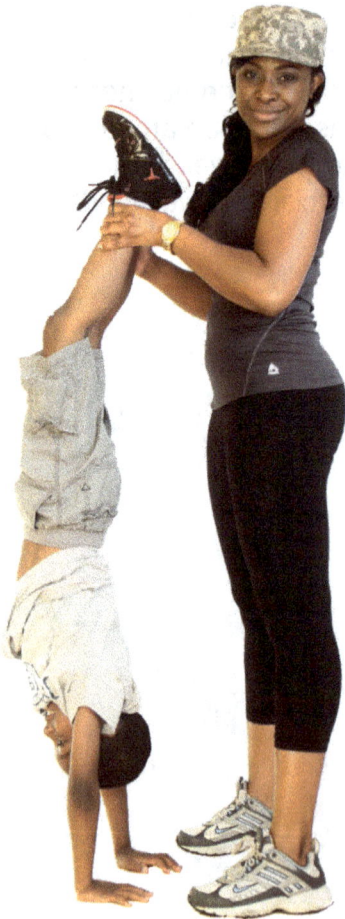

Grit Weinstein

Grit is the wife of the author, Colonel Weinstein. She is a registered nurse trained in Germany and worked for over 12 years as a nurse in Zurich, Switzerland where she was a research nurse in the area of spinal cord injuries and orthopedics. She is the author of several children's books.

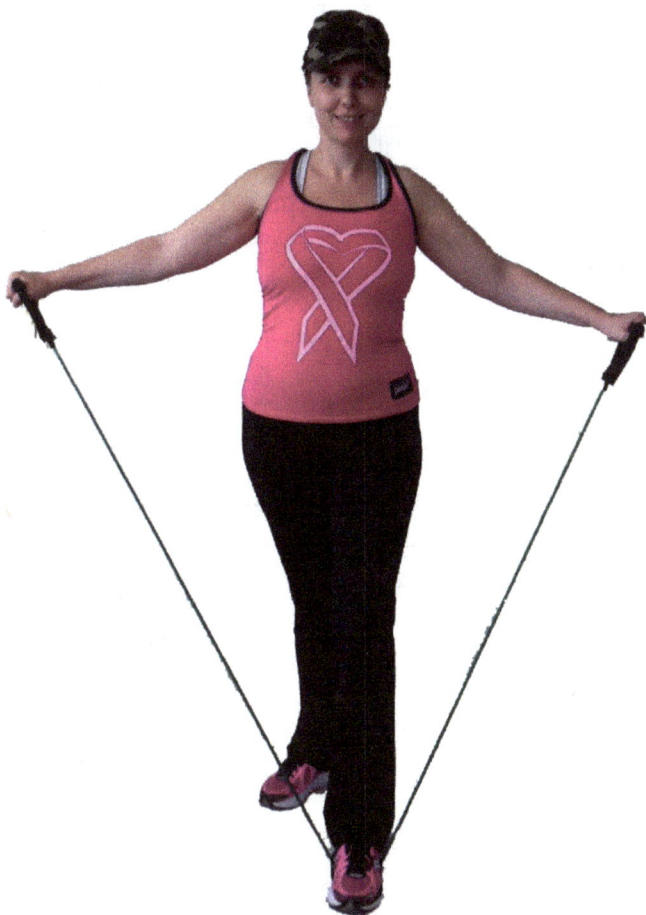

Day # _____

Your expectations decide your success.

Breakfast	Quantity	Calories	Fat grams	Carb grams	Protein grams	Fiber grams
Breakfast Totals						

Lunch	Quantity	Calories	Fat grams	Carb grams	Protein grams	Fiber grams
Lunch Totals						

Dinner	Quantity	Calories	Fat grams	Carb grams	Protein grams	Fiber grams
Dinner Totals						

M = Morning
A = Afternoon
E = Evening

Weight

Total 8 oz. glasses of water today:

Snacks	Quantity	Calories	Fat grams	Carbs grams	Protein grams	Fiber grams
Snack Totals						

Vitamins, Meds and other Supplements

		Calories	Fat grams	Carbs grams	Protein grams	Fiber grams
GRAND TOTALS > DAY#						

Physical Fitness

Type	Hours	Reps/Sets	Intensity	Calories Burned

	Bad									Excellent
My Attitude	1	2	3	4	5	6	7	8	9	10
On Track?	1	2	3	4	5	6	7	8	9	10
Belief Meter	1	2	3	4	5	6	7	8	9	10

"There are no hopeless situations, there are only people who have grown hopeless about them."
- Clare Boothe Luce

"He Ain't Heavy, He's My Brother."

The line "He ain't heavy, he's my brother," has been used for many decades now. That picture of one child carrying his or her brother is what comes to mind. Many artists have done versions of a song titled "He Ain't Heavy." There are so many fundraising events and activities to help animals, cancer research, diabetes research and many others. These are all worthy causes. What I have noticed is that our youth and children who are in need of help and guidance are not getting the same attention.

I have volunteered for the homeless and run-away children and have spoken with them about what they have experienced in life and how they got to where they are. It is not pretty. One kid responded to my question about how he came to the special home that was taking care of him. He responded, "My mother didn't want me." I had a hard time maintaining my composure as he was sharing his story with me. Why am I sharing this? I want to encourage you to donate time and / or money to help our youth, especially our troubled youth that need help getting back on track.

Here are some resources to help our youth:

The Covenant House
www.coveanthouse.org

Sheridan House
www.sheridanhouse.org

Books and Other Products by
Bob Weinstein
Lt. Colonel, U.S. Army, Ret.
www.BeachBootCamp.net

Boot Camp Fitness for All Shapes and Sizes
Paperback, ISBN 978-0-9841783-1-5
EBook, ISBN 978-0-984-17837-7 (all formats)

Boot Camp Six-Pack Abs
Paperback, ISBN 978-1-935759-17-1
EBook, 978-1-935759-19-5 (all formats)

600 Push-ups, 30 Variations
Paperback, ISBN 978-1-935759-09-6
EBook, ISBN 978-1-935759-10-2 (all formats)

Weight Loss - Twenty Pounds in Ten Weeks
Paperback, 220 pages, ISBN 978-0-9841783-0-8
EBook, ISBN 978-0-984-17834-6 (all formats)

Food & Fitness Journal
Paperback, ISBN 978-1-935759-03-4
EBook, ISBN 978-1-935759-05-8 (all formats)

Quotes, Wisdoms and Some Dumb Things
Paperback, ISBN 978-1-935759-11-9
EBook, ISBN 978-1-935759-15-7 (all formats)

Quotes to Live By
Paperback, ISBN 978-0-9841783-2-2
EBook, ISBN 978-0-984-17833-9 (all formats)

Discover Your Inner Strength (co-author)
Paperback, Ebook, ISBN 978-0-984-17836-0 (pdf)

Six Keys to Permanent Weight Loss
Audio book as MP3 download (Amazon), 60 minutes

Eight Secrets to Longevity, Health and Fitness
Audio book as MP3 download (Amazon), 50 minutes